MW00991914

UNLOCK THE POWER TO

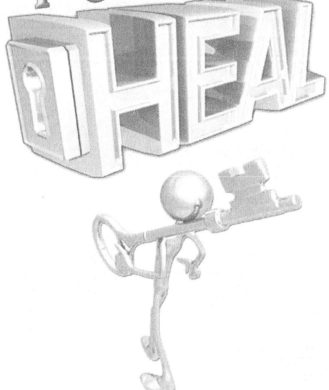

ROBERT SCOTT BELL
TY M. BOLLINGER

Printed and bound in the USA
ISBN 10: 0-9788065-4-9
ISBN 13: 978-0-9788065-4-5

To order more copies of this book,
please visit the following website:

www.UnlockThePowerToHeal.com

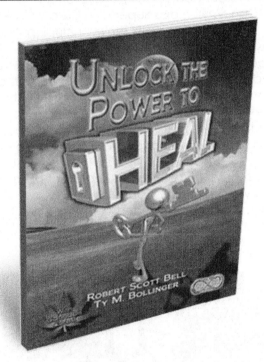

**Before you read this book, we must give you the
following FDA mandated warning and disclaimer:**

This book is for educational purposes only. It is not intended as a
substitute for the diagnosis, treatment, or advice of a qualified,
licensed medical professional. The facts presented in the following
pages are offered as information only, **not** medical advice.

The statements in this book have not been evaluated by the FDA
(the "Federal Death Administration"), the AMA ("American Murder
Association"), "Big Pharma," or the rest of the "Medical Mafia."

Vitamins K & G to the Super D

Heaping helpings of Vitamin K ("Kudos") and Vitamin G ("Gratitude") to our good buddy and producer of The Robert Scott Bell Show – Don Naylor, aka Super Don. Six days a week, Super Don brings the sound of The RSB Show, including "Outside the Box Wednesdays with Ty Bollinger," out to the world. Good vibrations don't happen by accident and Super Don wraps the spoken word of a talk radio show into production values as high as anything you will ever hear on multi-million dollar networks! He is the everyman with an ear to hear through the pharmaceutical cacophony of the mainstream media, so that we can put a healthy perspective on the news that would otherwise attempt to drug you to sleep.

Through the many years serving as producer of The RSB Show, Don has gone beyond the call of duty to see that our mission delivering health freedom and healing liberty continues despite all obstacles; hence, his most appropriate moniker, "Super Don!"

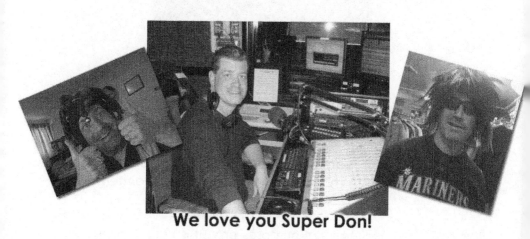

We love you Super Don!

Appreciation & Acknowledgements

~ *Robert Scott Bell*

My heartfelt gratitude goes to my wife Nancy for putting up with my long, self-imposed hours dedicated to bringing healing to all those ready to hear it (and now read it, too). I could not serve in this way without the patience, love and understanding and of course, all the delicious, nourishing, organic meals from my honey. She has given so much to make it possible to do all that I do, and I love her.

I am stoked that my awesome kids, Elijah and Ariana, have the benefit of learning in childhood that which I did not learn until after I had suffered 24 years of nutritional ignorance in my youth. Their spirit brings me great joy, even as they don't ask for permission when maybe it is required. Perhaps they listen too closely to my show. Or maybe it is because they are organic, unvaccinated and have not had to resort to antibiotics even once. May they be a shining light for the next generation.

Thanks to my mom, Miki Bell, who has put much of what I share in this book to the test and proved that it really works! She is 82 and takes no medications! It pays to listen to your son!

I am incredibly grateful for my friendship with Christopher Barr, whose commitment to whole food nutrition science has made accessible the oft overlooked basic tools for health recovery. Our shared respect and admiration for Antoine Béchamp drives us tirelessly to teach the "Law of the Terrain." He graciously shared his research on chromium, selenium and silica for your nutritional benefit.

I am truly grateful to fellow talk show host and friend Jerry Doyle from Epic Times, who continues to be a fearless defender of the information revealed within this book. From the first time that I appeared as a guest on The Jerry Doyle Show and revealed that in order to lose weight you have to eat more fat, he could have dismissed me as a crazy homeopath. Instead, he embraced the challenge and put my words to the test, even daring to drink whole milk instead of 2%. I only await the moment that he goes raw, too. While it would be much easier to dismiss ideas presented here that tend to poke the eye of established science, his keen intellect and willingness to question the status quo have brought many more people to realize that the power to heal is within their grasp. Thanks JD!

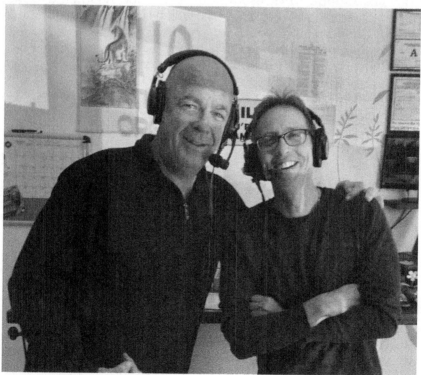
RSB and Jerry Doyle

I am profoundly grateful to Stephen Quinto, founder of Natural Immunogenics, for his miraculous breakthrough in hydrosol technology that allowed for the creation of a form of silver that has potency beyond compare while carrying the safety profile of a homeopathic remedy. Bioactive silver hydrosol is a unique species of silver that bridges the gap between the physical and energetic realms. This has made possible the use of the extraordinary properties of Argentum metallicum in entirely new ways.

I would like to acknowledge Dr. Eric Rentz, DO, CNMO, of the Project for Humanity, for his contributions to this silver-aloe healing protocol and for sharing his profound clinical experience in working with silver more comprehensively than any physician on the planet.

Also, special thanks to my good friend Ty Bollinger, without whom, I may never have gotten the first one published!

RSB and his family
Left to right - Ariana, Nancy, RSB, and Elijah

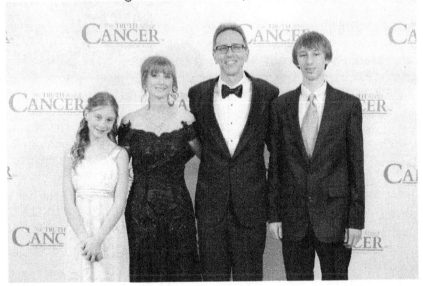

Appreciation & Acknowledgements

~ Ty Bollinger

My deepest thanks goes to my wonderful wife, Charlene, who is my "Princess" and my best friend. She spends countless hours educating our children, cooking delicious meals, keeping a peaceful home, and sacrifices in so many other ways that it would be impossible to list them all.

You've heard the phrase, *"Behind every great man there's a great woman."* Well, I'm not sure that "great" is a word that characterizes me, but it certainly does my wife. Thank you Sweetie! I love you, and always will.

To my four precious children, Brianna, Bryce, Tabitha, and Charity: *"Daddy loves you!"* I'm so thankful that you are growing up in a home that isn't afraid of the truth, no matter how uncomfortable it may be. Your desire for knowledge is encouraging to me and mommy. We pray that all four of you live your lives for Jesus.

And in today's toxic world, your mommy and daddy are so happy that you are learning how to stay healthy and help others get healthy too. So, keep on stepping **"outside the box"** in all areas of your lives and remember to do unto others as you would have them do unto you.

Thanks to Mom and Dad, who are both in Heaven with Jesus. They taught me to search for truth and to love others enough to share truth with them, even if they weren't "ready to hear it." In different ways, they were each my hero.

When I look back on my life, I can honestly say that I do not have a single bad memory of Mom and Dad. Their smiles were contagious, and so was their zest for life. Now that they are both gone, there are two holes in my heart which will never be filled. But I will see them both again in Heaven. That is my hope.

Lastly but not leastly (is that a word?), I want to thank my compadre and good friend, Robert Scott Bell. Teaming up with RSB these past several years has been awesome and I look forward to continuing to "rock the health world" with RSB for many years to come.

Charlene calls us the "dynamic duo," which is fine with me ... as long as I'm "Batman" and RSB is "Robin" (wearing the cute yellow cape with green tights).

TMB and his family
Left to right - Bryce, Charity, TMB, Charlene, Brianna & Tabitha

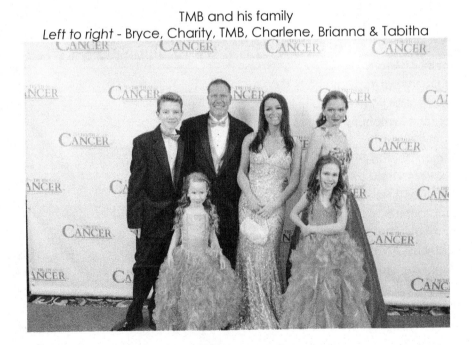

Table of Contents

Robert Scott Bell is a homeopathic practitioner with a passion for health and healing unmatched by anybody in media. Six days a week, Robert empowers his listeners with healing principles that can aid in physical, emotional, mental, spiritual, economic and yes, even political healing! The concept of nullification is a cornerstone of Robert's radio show where he reveals ways in which you can restore health without government interference or their permission.

On "The Robert Scott Bell Show," Robert hosts the fastest two hours of healing information on radio, dealing with everyday health issues from the perspective of alternative/holistic healthcare. He tackles the tough issues and shows no fear when confronting government and corporate bullies who would stand in the way of health freedom.

How does health freedom tie into the 10th Amendment? Robert says it is essential – without health freedom, the ability to defeat tyranny is doubly difficult. His message: "*Stop asking for permission where none is required.*"

His commentary crosses the political, economic and cultural divide, drawn from his 26 years of experience in the natural health care sector, whether providing direct support to those in need or working with physicians on their toughest cases. He makes sense out of medical propaganda, taking the complex and breaking it down into forms much easier to understand. His bottom line is bringing the freedom and power to heal back to the people, where it belongs.

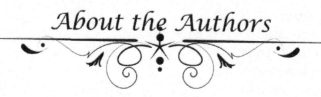

He personally overcame 24 years of chronic diseases using natural healing principles (without government permission) and has dedicated his life to revealing the healing power within all of us.

Learn more at www.RobertScottBell.com.

Ty Bollinger is a happily married husband and father, a CPA, health freedom advocate, health researcher, former competitive bodybuilder, talk radio host, documentary film producer, and best-selling author.

After losing several family members to cancer (including his mother and father), Ty refused to accept the notion that chemotherapy, radiation, and surgery (the "Big 3") were the most effective treatments available for cancer patients.

He began a quest to learn all he possibly could about alternative cancer treatments and the medical industry. What he uncovered was shocking: There is ample evidence to support the allegation that the "war on cancer" is largely a fraud and that multinational pharmaceutical companies are "running the show."

In 2014, Ty traveled the USA and interviewed the most renowned doctors and scientists about treating cancer naturally and eventually produced the documentary mini-series (docu-series) entitled *"The Quest for The Cures"* and *"The Quest for The Cures...Continues."* This docu-series was viewed by over 2 million people worldwide.

In 2015, Ty traveled the globe to interview more doctors, scientists, and cancer survivors and produced *"The Truth About Cancer: A Global Quest"* which aired in October 2015 and was viewed by over 5 million people worldwide.

Ty speaks frequently at conferences, expos, seminars, and churches and is a regular guest on multiple radio shows and writes for numerous magazines and websites. He also co-hosts "Outside the Box Wednesdays" on the "The Robert Scott Bell Show."

His websites are www.theTruthAboutCancer.com and www.CancerTruth.net.

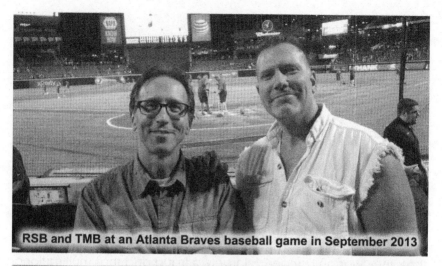

RSB and TMB at an Atlanta Braves baseball game in September 2013

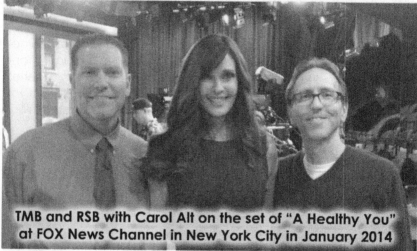

TMB and RSB with Carol Alt on the set of "A Healthy You" at FOX News Channel in New York City in January 2014

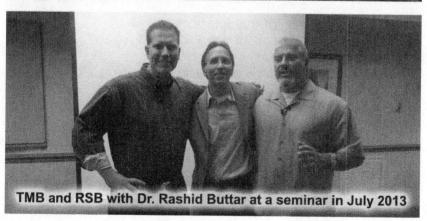

TMB and RSB with Dr. Rashid Buttar at a seminar in July 2013

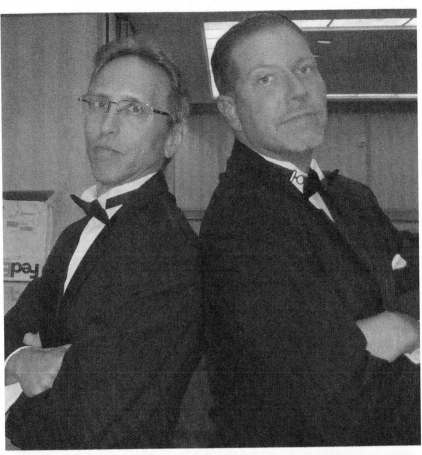

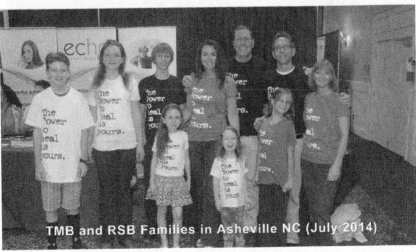

TMB and RSB Families in Asheville NC (July 2014)

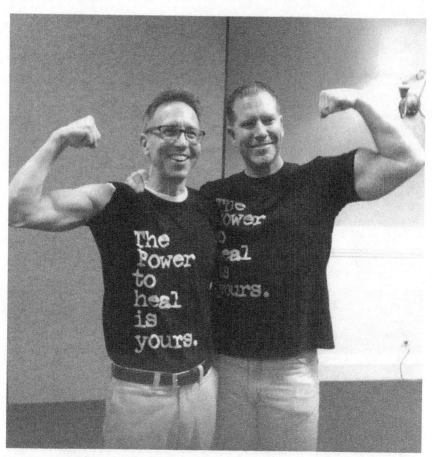

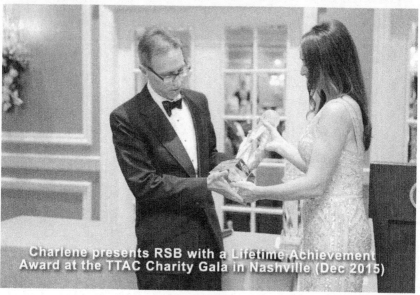

Charlene presents RSB with a Lifetime Achievement Award at the TTAC Charity Gala in Nashville (Dec 2015)

Introduction

Why did we write this book?

Because there is misconception about natural medicine in today's "Big Pharma" controlled world.

For much of our young lives, genuine healing was something out of reach, like it was locked away in a safe that we were unable to open. It can be both frustrating and frightening when you realize that the "experts" (medical doctors) know very little about accessing the natural tools for health recovery, much less health maintenance.

When that moment of disillusionment occurs, you have a choice to make. You can give up, because the authorities keep telling you that you can't possibly know how to heal yourself unless you have a degree and a license. Or you can recognize the truth that having a "duh"-gree or permission from the government can never replace your God-given birthright to do that which your cells know to be true.

But how do you get information that must be so valuable that it has been locked away and is seemingly unobtainable?

Easy ... ask TMB and RSB.

We wrote this book with the intention of providing you with keys necessary to **unlock the power to heal.**

By no means is this book a scholarly work. We decided to write this book in layman's terms, with a minimum of medical jargon and without long lists of references. Unlike Emeril Lagasse, who likes to "kick it up a notch," our goal was to "bring it down a notch" and enable you to actually comprehend the information about nutrition and overall health.

We both hope that you benefit from the book and that you are empowered with vital information which will allow you to **unlock the power to heal.**

18

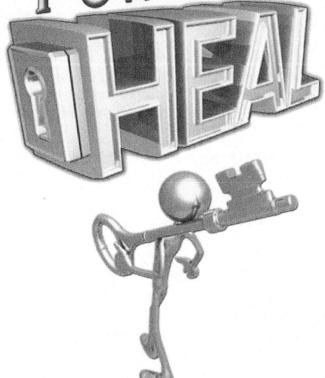

UNLOCK THE POWER TO HEAL

SECTION I

A Brief History

FLEXNER REPORT - FAUX PAS OR FRAUD?

The medical industry is nothing short of a *"Church of Pharmaceutical Mysticism"* with medical doctors the equivalent of *"high priests."* But modern medicine has only been around a little over 100 years, while traditional medical systems (such as Chinese and Ayurvedic medicine) have been in use for over 5,000 years.

Homeopathy has been in use for 200 years, chiropractic and naturopathic medicine have been utilized for over 100 years, and of course, people have been using herbs and dietary remedies since the beginning of recorded history.

The reality is that the M.D. "emperors" are buck naked. **Why do we say this?** In order to understand the current state of affairs of medical practice in the USA, it's vital to understand exactly how we got here. So, let's put on our history caps, jump into the time capsule, and go all the way back over 100 years to the turn of the 20th century.

Around 1900, the American Medical Association (AMA) was a weak organization with little money and little respect from the general public. Chiropractic had just been introduced into the mainstream, homeopathy was thriving, herbalists were flourishing, all the while regular doctors were unable to profit from their medical practices.

The AMA established a *Council on Medical Education* in 1904. This council's stated mission was to "upgrade medical education" – a noble goal. However, the *Council on Medical Education* had actually devised a plan to rank medical schools throughout the country, but their guidelines were dubious, to say the least. For instance, just having the word "homeopathic" in the name of a medical school reduced its ranking because the AMA asserted that such schools taught "an exclusive dogma."

However, by 1910, the AMA was out of money and didn't have the funds to complete the project. The Rockefellers had joined forces with the Carnegie foundation to create an education fund, and they were approached by N. P. Colwell (secretary of the *Council on Medical Education*) to finish the job they had started, but could no longer fund. Simon Flexner, who was on the Board of Directors for the Rockefeller Institute, proposed that his brother, Abraham, who knew nothing about medicine, be hired for the project. Rockefeller and Carnegie agreed.

Despite his lack of medical knowledge, the plan was to "restructure" the AMA and "certify" medical schools based solely

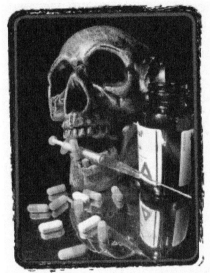

upon Flexner's recommendations. The AMA's head of the *Council on Medical Education* traveled with Flexner as they evaluated medical schools.

Eventually, Flexner submitted a report to The Carnegie Foundation entitled "Medical Education in the United States and Canada," which is also known as the "Flexner Report." Not surprisingly, the gist of the report was that it was far too easy to start a medical school and that most medical schools were not teaching "sound medicine."

Translation: they weren't pushing enough drugs (made by the companies owned by Carnegie and Rockefeller).

With the AMA grading the various medical colleges, it became predictable that the homeopathic colleges, even the large and respected ones, would eventually be forced to stop teaching homeopathy or die. That's exactly what happened. Published in 1910, the Flexner Report emphatically recommended the strengthening of medical courses in pharmacology (drugs) and the addition of research departments at all "qualified" medical schools.

With public backing secured by the publication of the Flexner Report, Carnegie and Rockefeller commenced a major upgrade in medical education by financing only those medical schools that taught what they wanted taught. In other words, they began to immediately shower many millions of dollars on those medical schools that were teaching "drug intensive" medicine.

Predictably, those schools that had the financing churned out the better doctors. In return for the financing, the schools were required to continue teaching course material that was exclusively drug oriented, with no emphasis put on natural medicine. The end result of the Flexner Report was that all accredited medical schools became heavily oriented toward drugs and drug research.

By 1925, over 10,000 herbalists were out of business. By 1940, over 1500 chiropractors would be prosecuted for practicing "quackery." The 22 homeopathic medical schools that flourished in 1900 dwindled to just 2 in 1923. By 1950, all schools teaching homeopathy were closed. In the end, if a physician did not graduate from a Flexner approved medical school and receive an M.D. degree, then he or she couldn't find a job.

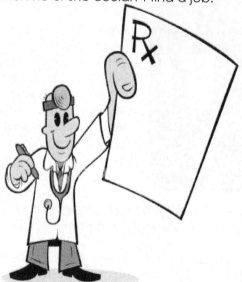

This is why today's M.D.s are so heavily biased toward synthetic drug therapy and know little about nutrition. They don't even study health; they study disease. Modern doctors are taught virtually nothing about nutrition, wellness or disease prevention. Expecting a medical doctor to guide you on health issues is sort of like expecting your CPA to pilot a jet airliner. It's simply **not** an area in which they have been trained.

A CENTURY OF PROGRESS?

Since the Flexner Report, have we seen progress? It's widely known that 100 years ago if a medical doctor saw a case of cancer he would call all his colleagues to come and have a look, telling them it was unlikely they would see another case, since cancer was so rare. Diabetes was practically unheard of, atherosclerosis was nonexistent, and the term "heart attack" hadn't even been coined yet. What did our great-grandfathers and great-grandmothers eat? Fresh vegetables, fresh fruits, bread from fresh grains, meat, butter, and cheese from grass-fed cows, and eggs from free-range chickens. None of it was processed with drugs and chemicals.

Today, cancer is an epidemic. According to the WHO in a 2010 study, 41% of the people alive today will face a diagnosis of the "Big C" (and that number was pre-Fukushima). Heart disease is rampant, and diabetes is endemic. Infant mortality is up; birth defects are up. Even closer to home, over 66% of American adults are overweight.

"Land of the Free, Home of the Obese"

Speaking of obesity, did you know that America is the most obese nation in the world? That's right. But the "good old USA" isn't just in first place, we're showboating in the end zone (with our twinkies and donuts) after an 85 yard TD pass! Being "obese" is categorized by having a body-mass index (BMI) greater than 30.

The top 5 most obese nations are:
#5 → Greece 22%
#4 → Slovack Republic 22%
#3 → UK 23%
#2 → Mexico 24%
... and your undisputed and still undefeated champion ... ... drum roll please ...
#1→ **USA 31%**

Yep, almost 1 in 3 Americans is con-sidered to be **OBESE!** A whopping 7% increase from the closest contender is pretty impressive, and that's coming from Mexico, a country that eats enchiladas, tacos, burritos, and nachos!

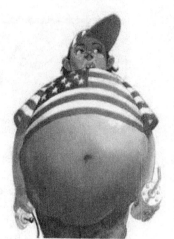

Here is a quote from a friend of mine who moved back to the USA after spending over a decade in Sweden. He emailed me his first day back in the USA after arriving in Kentucky.

"I was aware there was a problem with obesity in America for a few years, but until you are confronted face to fat face with so many huge fatties over and over in one day, well, it was very upsetting. Some people were so huge they could only waddle and limp along. So this is what 20 years of MSG and Aspartame addiction has caused, 200, 300, 400 pound people on the average. Even the people who are now considered to be average are 30 or 40 pounds overweight."

While we're on the subject of obesity, it's surprising how many people still believe that "diet" soda is a "good thing" for losing weight. In fact, we hear people all the time proudly state that they eat healthy and "only drink diet soda." So let's set the record straight; there is **nothing** even remotely healthy about drinking diet soda (specifically diet sodas sweetened with Aspartame). Even though diet sodas have zero calories, the artificial sweeteners (like Aspartame) tend to trigger more communication in the brain's "pleasure center" while not providing the brain with actual satisfaction.

According to Sharon Fowler, obesity researcher at UT Health Science Center at San Diego, *"Artificial sweeteners could have the effect of triggering appetite but unlike regular sugars they don't deliver something that will squelch the appetite."* Since your brain is not satisfied, the result is that you will crave **MORE** sugar, **MORE** carbs, and **MORE** calories. Result: Diet sodas will make you **FAT!** A recent 10 year study (of almost 500 diet soda drinkers) at the University of Texas showed that people who drink 2 or more

24

diet sodas per day had a 500% greater increase in waist size (compared to non-diet soda drinkers)!

So, not only is Aspartame [*formerly on a Pentagon list of biowarfare chemicals – until the FDA "approved" it for consumption*] an excitotoxin (i.e. it excites brain cells to death), and not only does it cause brain tumors, strokes, heart attacks, skin disorders, and seizures, but now we have proof that it actually makes you fatter!

Is that progress?

We spend **$1.5 trillion** per year for "health" care, most of which goes for administration and executive salaries.

- Who are the largest advertisers for TV and the printed media? **You got it! Big Pharma and Big Agra**.
- Do they want to keep the ball rolling? **Do fish swim?**
- Will they kill you to do it? **Is the pope Catholic?**
- Do they want people to take charge of their own health? **Negative Captain Kirk!**

We know this is depressing stuff, but don't give up just yet. It's important to explain exactly how we got here and what we can do about it.

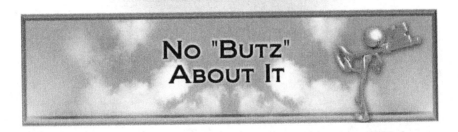

After World War II and the rise of the Industrial Revolution, agriculture in the USA was transformed dramatically, primarily due to the leadership of Secretary of Agriculture (Earl Butz) who told small farmers to **"*get big or get out.*"**

Mainstream farming became characterized by monoculture (growing a single crop for years and years), high yields, pesticides, fungicides, and mechanized tools, while "old timey" family farming based on biodiversity and generational knowledge was squeezed out.

And yes, as you might have guessed, farming became much more expensive for small farmers, thus forcing many to go into debt, or leave farming altogether.

Over the past half century, farming has been concentrated into the hands of a few powerful corporations (aka "Big Agra"). There are now fewer farms than ever before, but the size and power of Big Agra has grown immensely. As a matter of fact, upwards of 95% of the food in the USA is controlled by corporations which put **profits** before people.

Most Americans remain blissfully unaware (or just don't care) they are eating genetically modified organisms (GMOs) every day. In the past two decades, GMOs have completely infiltrated our farm fields, grocery stores, and kitchens to such an extent that most folks have no idea how many GMOs they actually consume daily.

If you haven't been paying attention to your food lately, Big Agra biotech giants (like MonSatan) thank you for that, because behind your back, they've successfully replaced over 90% of the corn and soy in the USA with their patented insecticide-producing "frankencorn" and "frankensoy."

If you ingest processed foods, bread, pasta, crackers, cake mixes, canola oil, mayonnaise, soymilk, veggie burgers, corn tortillas, corn chips, corn oil, corn syrup, or anything else made from corn, soy, or cotton, you are usually consuming GMOs. The first GMO food hit the market in 1994 (the "Flavr Savr" tomato). Since then, sugar beets, potatoes, corn, squash, rice, soybeans, vegetable oils and animal feed have all been manipulated. Each year, American farmers plant over 200 million acres of GMO crops. It is estimated that each person in the USA eats about 200 pounds of GMO foods per year!

We've let corporate interests turn us into poison-fed lab rats. And the foxes are now guarding the henhouse.

The proliferation of GMOs has corresponded with upticks in bowel diseases such as diverticulitis, colitis, and irritable bowel syndrome (IBS), Crohn's disease, leaky gut, and, especially in children, allergies.

Coincidence?

We don't think so. It's a massive human experiment, and we **all** are the guinea pigs.

Leaky gut syndrome takes place when fissures open between cells lining the gastrointestinal tract. Partially digested food particles ooze through those fissures into the body and appear to be foreign invaders. The immune system activates to do what it does best: **seek and destroy.** This is one of the main problems with GMOs – they introduce gene sequences that the body has never seen before. Our immune systems then attack the GMOs as if they were harmful pathogens (which they actually are).

Not only are GMOs in almost everything, but since labeling isn't required they remain hidden and you have to research all the potential ingredients that are likely to be GMO (which is also constantly increasing). Recent research has shown that GMOs are carcinogenic, toxic to the liver, kidneys, and blood.

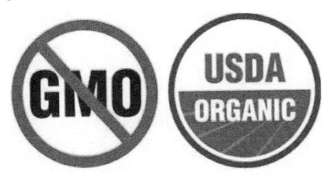

Now the question is this ... **are you going to sit back and accept this or are you going to do something about it?**

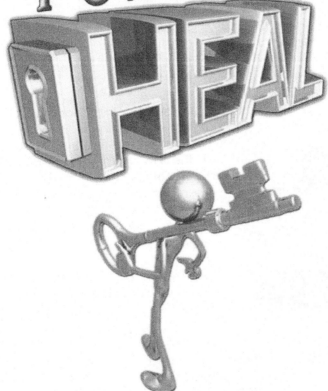

UNLOCK THE POWER TO HEAL

SECTION II
Key Issues & Micronutrients

SMOKE & MIRRORS

In today's world, relatively few people know how to maintain true health. Is this accidental or intentional? **You decide.**

What everyone **DOES** know is Coca Cola, hot dogs, Viagra, white bread, Big Macs, Whoppers, Ben & Jerry's, CVS Pharmacy, Tums, Pepto Bismol, and Vioxx. Oh yeah, and cheap, mass-produced, synthetic (chemical) grocery store vitamins.

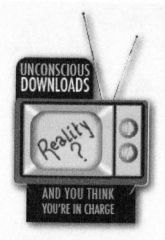

Control of information in America today is one of the most sophisticated systems of influence ever devised. This is the key to propaganda; people must **not** be taught how to think for themselves.

They must be conditioned to trust those in power and believe what they hear on TV and the radio. As a result, we have lost the ability to think logically for ourselves. We have become "dumb and dumber."

Interestingly, when we watch TV, activity in the higher brain regions (such as the neocortex) is diminished, while activity in the lower brain regions (such as the limbic system) increases. This basically means that we become "zombies" when we watch TV and are open to manipulation.

Another way to think of it is that we are opening ourselves to "unconscious downloads" when we sit and "veg" in front of the TV ... especially during the commercials.

You Are What You Eat

You are what you eat, right? Or, at least that is how the old adage goes. Yet, how many of us actually have a clue what we are eating? Where did your morning cereal come from? It was likely produced with GMO corn, GMO soy, and/or GMO sugar beets.

Ouch!

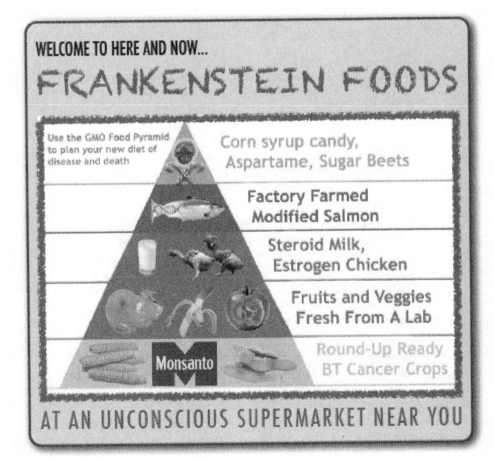

What about that yummy hamburger you just scarfed down after racing through the drive-through window at the local fast food joint? Ummmmmm, it was most likely from a cow raised in a CAFO (Concentrated Animal Feeding Operation), fed a GMO corn diet, and pumped full of rBGH and antibiotics. **Barf!**

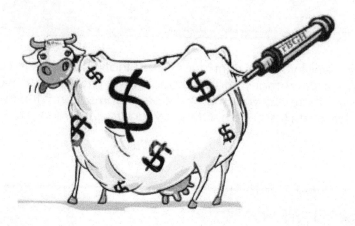

How many people actually eat organic, raw fruits and vegetables? How many families consume eggs from free range chickens and eat dairy products from organic, grass-fed cows or bison? Truth be told, processed, pesticide-laden, GMO food composes the majority of what most Americans eat. It's all marketing "smoke and mirrors" when you see certain buzz words. It is the art of persuading by suspending logic and twisting data into junk science.

Example: what's the actual difference in composition between Wheaties and Total, two cereals put out by the same company? Total is advertised as being much more nutrient-rich than "ordinary" Wheaties. Look at the labels. What justifies the extra $1.50 for a box of Total? Answer: a couple of pennies worth of synthetic vitamins sprayed over the Wheaties. That's it! That's what **"vitamin enriched"** means.

The other trick word is **"fortified."** Generally that means that the food itself is devoid of nutrients or enzymes, so they tried to pump it up a little with some "vitamins." Cheap synthetic vitamin sprays are all that is required for the manufacturer to use labels like "enriched" and "fortified." These words are red flags. If a food needs to be fortified or enriched, you can bet it was already dead.

THE STANDARD AMERICAN DIET IS "SAD"

The Standard American Diet ("SAD") typically consists of a myriad of processed carbs (cereals, breads, pasta, cookies, cakes, etc.), processed meat products, and a few fruits and veggies. The "SAD" is high in many things, most of which your body doesn't really need, including GMO high fructose corn syrup, hydrogenated oils, MSG, GMO soy, and sodium nitrate.

Glaringly absent are essentials such as vitamins and minerals.

Surgeon General's

WARNING:

The Standard American Diet causes approximately 2/3 of the deaths due to disease in America.

It's a fact, folks. Most people eating the "SAD" are deficient in vitamins and minerals. Some of the common deficiencies have major consequences.

For instance, vitamin B12 deficiency (associated with low stomach acid) causes severe neurological injury which is often irreversible; folic acid (actually folate) deficiency greatly increases the risk of birth defects and adult male heart attacks; selenium deficiency can impact the thyroid and lead to hypothyroidism.

A major problem today is poor food choices. A recent survey indicated that fruits and vegetables comprise only 7% of the average American's diet. Wow! Can anyone say, "Malnourished"? If you're eating primarily processed foods and pasteurized dairy products, you're not getting the vitamins and minerals you need from your food.

Vitamins and minerals are particularly important for persons with environmental illness, who are sick because their detoxification systems have been overwhelmed. Many vitamins and minerals are "cofactors" for the various detoxification enzymes, and get depleted when the body's system has a lot of work to do. The term "coenzyme" is oftentimes used to describe vitamins that function as cofactors.

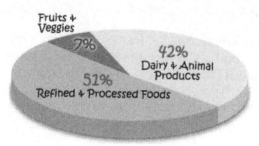

Fruits & Veggies 7%

42% Dairy & Animal Products

51% Refined & Processed Foods

Basically, a cofactor is a chemical compound that is required for certain enzymes (called conjugated enzymes) to become active. Cofactors, vitamins, and minerals help bodies function properly, they can boost the immune system, they support normal growth and development, and they help cells and organs function properly.

Vitamins, cofactors, and minerals have a fundamental role in cellular energy generation or metabolism. They are necessary in numerous metabolic processes and are active proton and electron carriers in the ATP-generating cellular respiratory chain.

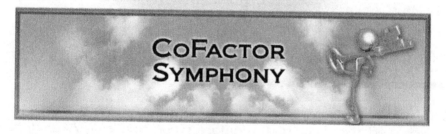

COFACTOR SYMPHONY

Did you know that most of us are at risk for mineral deficiency disease (MDD) since minerals are conspicuously absent from our soils? Did you know that there is not a mineral in this world (or any essential nutrient, for that matter) able to confer benefit **in isolation?**

Minerals work in tandem with vitamins and with fatty acids and particularly in tandem with macronutrients like protein, carbohydrates, and fiber. Simply put, they make each other work. Mineral deficiencies can cause vitamin deficiencies, and vice versa. They work in harmony, like a well-orchestrated symphony.

A perfect example of this is calcium. It's generally accepted that we need calcium to build and maintain strong bones and teeth and joints. But supplementing with calcium **alone** does more harm than good. Without magnesium, vitamin D, zinc, boron **and** high quality, bioavailable protein, our bodies do not know what to do with the calcium.

Without these "cofactors," the body's tissue literally chokes on the calcium, sort of like filling an engine with gasoline but forgetting to give it oxygen. **Gag! Choke!** Flooded engine. In the case of calcium, without the co-factors, it gets deposited in tissue (known as "calcification") and is one of the signs of aging. Eventually it can cause premature death. Quite literally, we turn to stone.

Let's go back to the engine example. What happens if we mix a little air with the gasoline? **Boom!** ... The engine ignites!

Voila! Similarly, if we mix in zinc, vitamin D, magnesium, silicon, boron and **protein** with the calcium, then the body understands what's going on, the cells turn on, and the body begins to function at optimal levels.

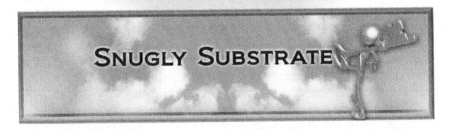

SNUGLY SUBSTRATE

Enzymes coordinate the millions of chemical reactions that happen in our cells each and every day. Every enzyme is in charge of one reaction, and for that reaction to happen, the substance involved has to fit in a little nook in the enzyme.

The nook is called the enzyme's active site, and it contains the perfect shape and charge for the reacting substance (**the substrate**) to fit in snugly. Some enzymes have active sites that are ready to go, but others need to get a slight "tweak" in their shape so they can get a firm hold on the substrate, forming a snugly enzyme-substrate complex.

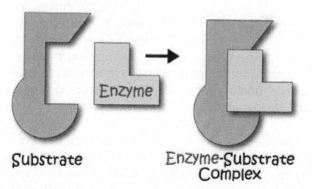

Substrate   Enzyme-Substrate Complex

And that's where cofactors (vitamins and minerals) appear. When a cofactor binds to an enzyme it changes the shape of the active site so it's just the right fit for the substrate.

Vitamin C is an excellent example of a cofactor that helps "tweak" the enzyme's active site. As you probably know (you **do** know this, don't you?), vitamin C is essential for the formation of collagen, a protein that acts like fiberglass reinforcement for our bodies. Collagen keeps our skin firm, forms the scabby scaffolding that new skin grows on after we're wounded, and helps keep our organs in one place rather than sloshing around our bodies.

The key to collagen's strength is its shape. It's made up of fibers twisted together like rope. A bunch of enzymes are involved in making and twisting collagen, and one of those enzymes needs a molecule of vitamin C to do its job. The vitamin C locks onto the enzyme's active site, changing its shape so it's a snug fit for the collagen molecule (substrate). The enzyme makes a chemical modification in the collagen to facilitate the snug fit we need.

Without vitamin C, the enzyme can't get a hold on the collagen, and the resulting fibers come out a little frayed. Without top notch collagen, our wounds don't heal properly, giving us gums and complexions that only a mother could love.

DOCTOR, DOCTOR, GIMME SOME NEWS

When a doctor says that supplements are all superfluous because we can get everything we need from our food, that doctor is ignorant of rudimentary information published and agreed upon by his own peers.

Whether or not we need supplementation is no longer an issue. The issue is **what kind** and **how much**. It's safe to say that vitamin and mineral deficiency can be linked to practically **any** disease syndrome known to man.

The problem is that the overwhelming majority of over-the-counter vitamins and minerals either do not contain what they claim to contain, or contain it in a biologically inactive form, or contain a combination of toxic, synthesized chemicals.

Most vitamins cannot be made by the body; they must be ingested. Obviously, the best sources are whole foods, which are rich in vitamins and minerals, right?

Well, maybe ... Sort of ...

Due to air pollution, soil depletion, mineral depletion, pesticides, insecticides, herbicides, and fungicides (The term "cide" means "being killed"), the fruits, vegetables, and grains grown in American soil today have only a fraction of the nutrient value they had in 1900.

The following excerpts concerning Senate Document 264 of the 74th Congress, 2nd Session 1936, were found in the March 1936 issue of Cosmopolitan: "... *99 percent of the American people are deficient in ... minerals, and ... a marked deficiency in any one of the more important minerals actually results in disease.*"

37

Folks, this was in 1936. Just think about the farming practices we employ today.

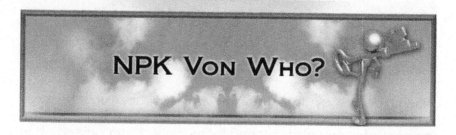

NPK Von Who?

Following the German agricultural methods of Justus von Liebig in the mid-1800s, American farmers found that N-P-K (nitrogen, phosphorus, and potassium) was all that was necessary for crops to **look good.** As long as N-P-K is added to the soil, crops can be produced and sold year after year from the same soil. Kind of like a mannequin in the window, they "look" good, but they're empty inside. The trace minerals vital for human nutrition are virtually absent from most American soil after all these years.

Von Liebig was responsible for the theory that N-P-K levels are the basis for determining healthy plant growth. However, this theory doesn't take into account the dozens of other nutrients and elements that are essential to plant growth such as sulfur, hydrogen, oxygen, carbon, magnesium, etc.

Nor does the theory include the importance of beneficial soil-based organisms (SBO) that help plants flourish and fight off pests and diseases. Additional nutrients such as carbon, hydrogen, oxygen, sulfur, magnesium, copper, cobalt, sodium, boron, molybdenum, and zinc are just as important to plant development as N-P-K.

As previously discussed (you didn't forget did you?), many of these minerals (such as zinc, copper, and magnesium) are necessary cofactors of vitamin activity.

Thus, it becomes painstakingly clear that supplementation is **vital.**

"BUT I DON'T NEED NO STINKING SUPPLEMENTS!"

Yes you do! Remember, the foods you eat have been stripped of most of their nutrients due to poor soil and from the process that refines and manufactures them. Most foods on the grocery store shelves are chock-full of unhealthy (trans) fats, refined sugars, refined salt, and are almost completely devoid of any nutritional value. Adding insult to injury, many foods today contain pesticides, fungicides, sulfites, and other preservatives.

You see, folks, Big Agra has one motive: **profit.**

Such a focus has resulted in an output of empty produce and a nation of unhealthy people. **The earth's immune system is its soil.** To be vital and capable of growing vital foods, soil must be rich in both minerals and soil-based organisms (SBOs).

But as we've already mentioned, the foods grown in American soil have only a fraction of the nutrients that were present a half century ago. Throw in the facts that most of our foods today are highly processed, genetically modified, and prepared in a way

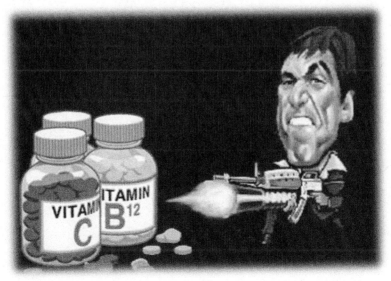

that often destroys much of the nutritional content, we've got a real problem, don't we?

To add insult to injury, it's not how much you eat; it's how much you **digest**. In other words, if our digestive systems functioned optimally, we wouldn't need as many high-quality nutrients in supplement form. However, that is not the case. Antibiotics have killed the beneficial bacteria in our guts, and we're in bad shape. So, we must go ...

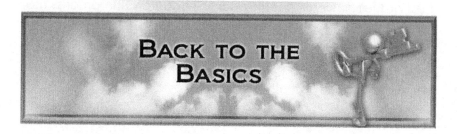

BACK TO THE BASICS

OK, OK, we know, we know. You want us to define some terms. **No problemo.**

Each and every day your body produces skin, muscle, and bone. It churns out rich red blood cells that carry nutrients and oxygen to remote outposts, and it sends nerve signals skipping along thousands of miles of brain and body pathways. It also formulates chemical messengers that shuttle from one organ to another, issuing the instructions that help sustain your life.

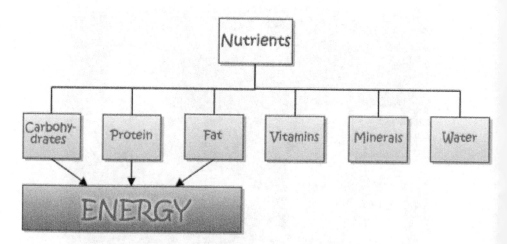

To do all this, your body requires some raw materials (nutrients), but trying to keep track of what all these nutrients do can be confusing. Read enough articles on the topic, and your eyes may swim with the alphabet-soup references to these nutrients, which are known mainly by their initials (such as vitamins A,B,C,D,E, and K—to name just a few).

There are six nutrient groups – water, vitamins, minerals, fats, proteins, and carbohydrates. All six groups are necessary for optimal health. The 3 **macronutrients** of protein, fat, and carbohydrates all perform essential roles in the human body. Our bodies require other nutrients as well, such as vitamins and minerals. However, these are needed in much smaller quantities, and thus are referred to as **micronutrients.**

MICTONUTRIENTS DE-"MYSTIFIED"

Vitamins and minerals are often called micronutrients because your body needs only tiny amounts of them. Yet failing to get even those small quantities virtually guarantees disease. Here are a few examples of diseases that can result from vitamin deficiencies:

- **Scurvy.** Old-time sailors learned that living for months without fresh fruits or vegetables (the main sources of vitamin C) causes the bleeding gums and lethargy associated with scurvy.
- **Blindness.** In some developing countries, people still become blind from vitamin A deficiency.
- **Rickets.** A deficiency in vitamin D can cause rickets, a condition marked by soft, weak bones that can lead to skeletal deformities such as bowed legs.

Just as a lack of key micronutrients can cause substantial harm to your body, getting sufficient quantities can provide a substantial benefit. Some examples of these benefits:

- **Strong bones.** A combination of calcium, vitamin D, vitamin K, magnesium, silicon, and phosphorus protects your bones against fractures.
- **Prevents birth defects.** Taking folate supplements (avoid synthetic folic acid) early in pregnancy helps prevent brain and spinal birth defects in offspring.

Many micronutrients interact. For instance, vitamin D enables your body to pluck calcium from food sources passing through your digestive tract rather than harvesting it from your bones. Vitamin C helps you absorb iron. However, the interplay of micronutrients isn't always cooperative. For example, vitamin C blocks your body's ability to assimilate the essential mineral copper, and even a minor overload of the mineral manganese can worsen iron deficiency.

Just to clarify.... many people think minerals and vitamins are the same, but they are not. The main difference is that vitamins are organic substances (meaning that they contain the element carbon) and can be broken down by heat, air, or acid, whereas minerals are **in**organic substances that hold on to their chemical structure.

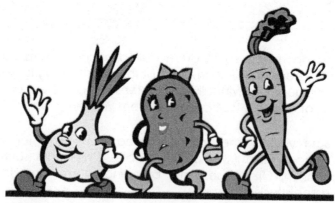

So why does this matter? It means the minerals in soil and water easily find their way into your body through the plants, fish, animals, and fluids you consume. But it's tougher to shuttle vitamins from food and other sources into your body because cooking, storage, and simple exposure to air can inactivate these more fragile compounds.

VITAMINS – A VESTIGE OF THE VOX POPULI

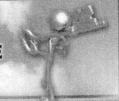

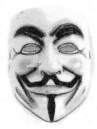

Voilà! Verily, verily, whether you are a victim or villain, and whether you are venal, vicious, virulent, or valiant and full of valor, the fact is that vitamins are vital, complex chemical elements that should never be vanquished. They enable the body to break down and use the basic elements of food, proteins, carbohydrates and fats.

Certain vitamins are also involved in producing blood cells, hormones, genetic material and chemicals in your nervous system. Unlike carbohydrates, proteins and fats, vitamins and minerals do not provide calories. However, they do help the body to use the energy from food. Most vitamins cannot be made in your body, so they must be acquired from food. One exception is vitamin D, which is made in the skin when it is exposed to sunlight. Bacteria present in the gut can also make some vitamins.

You might think of how vitamins help you at the current moment, but vitamins played a role in your life before you were even born. Folic acid (use the folate form only) and whole food chromium help to prevent birth defects. Again, going back to the time of conception until now, some vitamins and minerals such as calcium, iron and vitamin D have played a crucial role in working together to form and maintain your bones and help them grow. As you age, they will become even more important as your skeletal system may falter as regenerative processes diminish and the demand for these vitamins and minerals increases.

Vitamins are either **water-soluble** or **fat-soluble**. Water soluble vitamins can be dissolved in water and are found in non-fatty, water-based food such as fruit and vegetables. They are absorbed directly into the bloodstream as food is broken down during digestion or as a supplement dissolves. Because much of your body consists of water, many of the water-soluble vitamins circulate easily in your body. Your kidneys continuously regulate levels of water-soluble vitamins, shunting excesses out of the body in your urine.

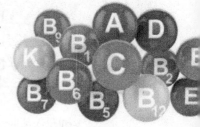

Fat-soluble vitamins are found in fatty foods and as their name suggests, they can be dissolved in fat. But rather than slipping easily into the bloodstream like most water-soluble vitamins, fat-soluble vitamins gain entry to the blood via lymph channels in the intestinal wall. Many fat-soluble vitamins travel through the body only under escort by proteins that act as carriers.

There are **four** fat-soluble vitamins [*vitamins A, D, E and K*] and **ten** water-soluble vitamins [*vitamin C, choline, and the eight B vitamins: biotin, thiamin (B1), riboflavin (B2), niacin (B3), pantothenic acid (B5), pyridoxine (B6), folic acid/folate (B9) and cobalamin (B12)*].

MAGNIFICENT MAJESTIC MINERALS

Four elements compose 96% of the body's makeup: carbon, hydrogen, oxygen, and nitrogen. The remaining 4% of the body's composition is minerals. Minerals are chemical elements that are involved in various processes in your body. They help to regulate

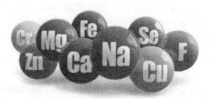

cell function and to serve as building blocks for your cells and organs. Unlike vitamins, minerals do not deteriorate during storage or cooking. There are several opinions about how many minerals are essential. Some say 14, some say 16, the debate is ongoing, kind of like how many angels can fit on the head of a pin. Does it really matter?

Anyway, at least everyone is in agreement that we all need small amounts of about 25-30 minerals (14-16 of which are considered to be "essential") to maintain normal body function and good health, but (as we've already mentioned) due to unwholesome dietary habits and also poor soil conditions, most of us are mineral deficient. It is interesting to note that unrefined sea salt and ancient mineral crystal salts contain 74-84 trace elements.

There are two groups of minerals: **macrominerals** (aka "major minerals") and **microminerals** (aka "trace minerals").

Macrominerals are needed in the diet in amounts of 100 milligrams or more each day. They include potassium, chlorine, phosphorus, calcium, magnesium, sulfur, and sodium. Macrominerals are present in virtually all cells of the body. They maintain general homeostasis and are required for normal functioning.

Microminerals include iron, copper, fluoride, molybdenum, chromium, manganese, iodine, zinc, and selenium. They are dietary minerals needed by the human body in very small quantities as opposed to macrominerals which are required in larger quantities.

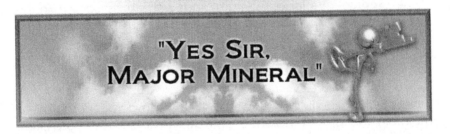

The body needs (and stores) relatively significant quantities of the major minerals. But those major minerals don't need to get a big head! They are no more significant to your health than the trace minerals; they're just present in your body in larger quantities.

Major minerals travel through the body in multiple methods. For instance, calcium acts like a fat-soluble vitamin because it requires a carrier for absorption and transport.

However, potassium acts more like a water-soluble vitamin since it is quickly absorbed into the bloodstream where it circulates freely and is excreted by the kidneys.

Speaking of potassium...

When you pick up a glass of water, your brain sends signals (electrical impulses) to your hand to tell it to grip the glass and bring it to your mouth. Breathing and blinking also require electrical impulses, but these are involuntary actions. Your brain tells your body when to breathe, when to blink, and when to pick up your foot while walking. Potassium helps conduct these electrical impulses.

Beware soldier!

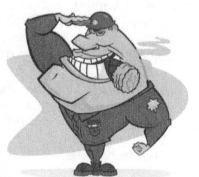

Having too much of one major mineral can result in a deficiency of another. These sorts of imbalances are usually caused by overloads from supplements, not food sources.

Here are two examples:

- **Sodium overload.** Calcium binds with excess sodium in the body and is excreted when the body senses that sodium levels must be lowered.
- **Excess phosphorus.** Too much phosphorus can hamper your ability to absorb magnesium.

One of the significant responsibilities of macrominerals is to maintain the proper balance of water in the body. Potassium, chloride, and sodium lead the charge in doing this. Sulfur helps stabilize protein structures, including some of those that make up hair, skin, and nails. Calcium, magnesium, silicon, and phosphorus are imperative for healthy bones.

THEY VANISHED WITHOUT A TRACE (MINERAL)

A thimble could easily contain the concentration of all the trace minerals ideally found in your body. Yet their contributions are just as critical as those of major minerals such as calcium and phosphorus, which each account for more than a pound of your body weight.

Trace minerals include chromium, selenium, zinc, manganese, molybdenum, iron, fluoride, iodine, and copper. Trace minerals carry out a diverse set of tasks.

Here are a few examples:

- **Zinc** helps blood clot, is essential for taste and smell, and bolsters the immune response.
- **Iron** is a critical component of hemoglobin in the red blood cells.
- **Copper** helps form several enzymes, one of which assists with iron metabolism and the creation of hemoglobin, which carries oxygen in the blood.

Trace minerals interact with one another, sometimes in ways that can trigger imbalances. Too much of one can cause or contribute to a deficiency of another. For example, a minor overload of manganese can exacerbate iron deficiency. When the body has too little iodine, thyroid hormone production slows, causing sluggishness and weight gain as well as other health concerns. The problem worsens if the body also has too little selenium.

Remember, with minerals, more is not necessarily better. Excessive intake of a dietary mineral may lead to illness either directly or indirectly because of the competitive nature between mineral levels in the body.

VIRTUAL REALITY, JUMBO SHRIMP, & SYNTHETIC VITAMINS

What do all of these phrases have in common? **They are all oxymorons!** No, we're not saying that they are "morons," they're **OXY**morons, which simply means that they are apparent contradictions.

Wholefood vitamins are increasing in popularity as people are recognizing that vitamins derived from wholefoods are often different from the synthetic (chemical) vitamins prepared in factories.

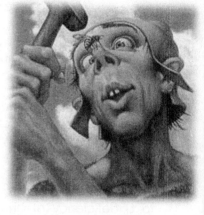

If you are one of those people taking over-the-counter synthetic vitamins, you may not be getting the quantity or quality of vitamins you thought you were getting. In fact, most easily available multivitamins are manufactured by one or more of the Big Pharma chemical companies.

The preparation of synthetic vitamins involves making a molecule that is one component of a large wholefood molecule. The wholefood vitamin is complete with the cofactors and other components needed to help the vitamin do its job. Because they are not complete, synthetic vitamins may actually work more like a drug, if they work at all, rather than as nutrients derived from real food.

UNLOCK THE POWER TO HEAL

SECTION III
Some Successful Solutions

FRIENDLY FLORA: "THE GOOD GUYS"

Probiotic consists of "pro" (supporting or favoring) and "biotic" (pertaining to life or specific life conditions).

"**Probiotics**" are micro-organisms, specific bacteria, fungi and yeasts that are a natural, necessary, component of the digestive

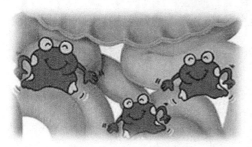

tract. Before we were born, our digestive tracts were void or empty of any bacteria. But we all get a mouthful of bacteria when we come through the birth canal; then during the first few weeks of life, breast-feeding establishes a base of "friendly flora" that coats the entire tract. These "good guys" will fight off and act as a defense against any harmful pathogens and bacteria ("bad guys"). By the time we reach adulthood, we will have approximately 3½ pounds of bacteria (this includes both good guys and bad guys) in our intestines.

As long as the good guys flourish, they keep you healthy by naturally boosting the immune system. They produce natural antibiotics that inhibit the growth and activity of the bad guys, while increasing the body's production of gamma interferon (an important antiviral molecule made by T-cells) and increasing enzyme production such as proteases and lipases. However, if our intestinal environment is disrupted, pathogenic bacteria, fungi, and parasites move in, multiply, and attack the beneficial bacteria. Unfortunately, as we age (actually, get more toxic and nutrient deficient), the good guys die off, so it's vital for us to replenish these "friendly flora" if we want to maintain the health of our digestive tract.

Beware! Anyone who has ever taken a round of **antibiotics** should realize that antibiotics destroy the good guys as well as the bad guys! Probiotics re-colonize symbiotic gut bacteria in healthy new terrain (microbiome). We recommend Dr. Ohhira's Probiotics (2 per night) while on the silver-aloe protocol (discussed later in the book). Then take 2 tablets, 3 times per day for two weeks once the silver-aloe protocol is complete.

STUPENDOUS SELENIUM

Remember the section on our "SAD" diet? Well, according to a US government survey a few years ago, the #1 food consumed by Americans is refined, bleached white flour. The whole grains that are refined to this white flour (aka "white death") are one of the highest sources of **selenium**. However, over 90% of the selenium is removed by the rendering of whole grains into refined, bleached white flour.

Consider also that the selenium content of foods has been greatly reduced over the past 100 years because of changes in farming practices over that period of time. Brazil nuts once contained 800 micrograms of selenium per 100 gram portion (almost 4 ounces). Recent assays show little more than 100 micrograms in the same quantity. Then consider that no other food even approaches even that level of selenium and you'll realize that supplementation is a necessity.

It was determined in the year 2000 that foods in America contain significantly less selenium than measured in previous decades. The Institute of Medicine that advises the federal government responded to this **not** with alarm at the great reduction but rather suggested **reducing** the previous recommendation of 200 micrograms daily consumption to just 55 micrograms daily. That is less than 10% of the high end consumption of Japanese on a traditional diet who coincidentally have the lowest cancer rate and greatest longevity in the world.

It was not until 1949 that selenium was first noted as a cancer preventative by Doctors Clayton and Baumann in the journal *Cancer Research*. Since then, selenium has been shown in multiple studies to be an effective tool in warding off various types of cancer, including breast, esophageal, stomach, prostate, liver, and bladder cancers. The scientific and medical literature is filled with studies that demonstrate selenium's anticancer effects in humans. As a matter of fact, the effectiveness of selenium as a cancer preventative has been demonstrated greater than any other substance ever tested whether medical, nutritional, herbal or any other.

For example, in an epidemiological study, Dr. Raymond Shamberger categorized the states and cities in the USA according to whether there was high, medium, or low selenium availability in the diet. He demonstrated an inverse association between selenium availability and age-adjusted mortality for all types of cancer. To put it simply, **the more selenium available, the lower the levels of cancer.**

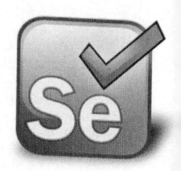

In a worldwide study Dr. Gerhard Schrauzer, M.D., Ph.D. (professor of medical chemistry at the University of California at San Diego) analyzed the blood-bank data from 27 countries around the world. He compiled a list in order of their blood selenium levels disclosing an inverse proportional relationship to cancer incidence, reporting specifically that areas with low levels of selenium in the diet had higher levels of leukemia and cancers of the breast, colon, rectum, prostate, ovary, and lung. In other words, the number one nation in blood selenium level (Japan) had the lowest cancer level (and consistently has rated highest in longevity) while the number two selenium level nation had the second lowest cancer rate, etc. etc.

Selenium was initially used in conventional medicine as a treatment for dandruff, but our comprehension of the mineral has dramatically increased over the past 20 years. It is an essential component of a powerful antioxidant manufactured by the body. This antioxidant, called glutathione peroxidase, defends specifically against peroxides, a type of free radical that attacks fats. Like other antioxidants, glutathione peroxidase also reduces the risk of developing cancer and heart diseases and stimulates the immune system's response to infections. This important enzyme is selenium dependent, with each molecule of the enzyme containing four atoms of selenium.

Research shows selenium (especially when used in conjunction with vitamins C, E, and beta-carotene) works to block many chemical reactions that create free radicals in the body. Remember, free radicals can damage our cellular DNA, which eventually can lead to degenerative diseases like cancer. Selenium also helps to prevent damaged DNA molecules from reproducing and proliferating, a process called mitosis. In other words, selenium acts to prevent tumors from developing.

Medical studies of chemotherapy (comparing those who also take selenium to those who do not) consistently find better results in those taking selenium with chemotherapy as to those taking chemo alone. Additionally, selenium protects against the damaging effects of radiation. Increased selenium intake boosts immune system function facilitating improved healing so that recovery from surgical procedures is enhanced. In other words, increased selenium is not only a beneficial option for prevention of cancer, but it can also be effective as a treatment option and as an effective adjunct to the "Big 3" (chemotherapy, radiation and surgery).

Our good friend, attorney Jonathan Emord, has taken the FDA to court on the matter of allowing label claims stating that selenium may prevent cancer. He has prevailed against the FDA in federal court more than half a dozen times on the matter of selenium. No other attorney has defeated the FDA in court more times than Emord so that he has earned the honorable title of "FDA dragonslayer."

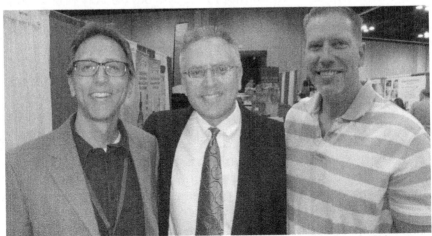

RSB, Jonathan Emord, and TMB at the 2013 Health Freedom Expo in Chicago

The old expression is *"an ounce of prevention is worth a pound of cure."* It would take almost 100 years at almost 800 mcg daily of selenium to consume a pound. Only 200 mcg daily supplementation of selenium has been documented to dramatically reduce cancer incidence, when in a grown, food-formed variety.

A daily intake of 400 mcg was recommended by Dr. Schrauzer, mentioned earlier in this article. A daily intake of 600 mcg has been documented for residents of Japan on a traditional Japanese diet where cancer incidence is lowest and longevity is the greatest in the world. If every man, woman, and child supplemented with 200 mcg of selenium, we could almost wipe out the cancer epidemic over night!

There is no downside to selenium supplementation, except perhaps to Big Pharma and the Medical Mafia, as this would definitely cut into their revenue streams!

THE SAD, SULLEN SAGA OF SELENIUM SLANDER

Tragically, peppered throughout this selenium century has been a consistent backlash about toxicity with selenium in what our friend, Chris Barr, often refers to as the *"sad, sullen saga of selenium slander."*

Whether addressing those claims from a medical or nutritional background about selenium benefits, there is an almost universal "selenium can be toxic" catchphrase that pervades medical "wisdom" (is that another oxymoron?).

Is selenium toxic? Heck, oxygen can be deadly in a variety of ways (depending upon amount and form) yet neither of us has ever heard a warning about "not breathing too deeply" or admonishments to "only breathe shallowly," both of which seem patently absurd.

So it is with selenium and in fact there is an important interplay between oxygen and selenium. Selenium is exceedingly important to offset damaging effects of normal oxygen metabolism within the body. In fact, there are far more documented cases of damage from therapeutic oxygen than there are of ill effects from selenium intake. Oxygen in the air we breathe is the best and safest form of oxygen. In a similar manner selenium compounds formed in the growth processes of food are also the best and safest forms.

Selenium toxicity is determined by the accumulation of selenium in the system if the body is unable to utilize it. That is why only the highest quality selenium supplementation should be utilized. Grown, wholefood varieties of selenium have been documented to offer the highest bioavailability and activity within the body and are the least likely to reach toxic levels. That is because they are utilized by the body so as not to accumulate in the body from nonusage.

Both of our families take "Innate Response" selenium at www.choosetobehealthy.com, recommended by our friend, Chris Barr. Much of this section on selenium was excerpted (with permission) from his booklet about selenium.

"ON YOUR MARK ... GET SET ... CHROMIUM!"

The mineral **chromium** is important from the very earliest stage of life; witness to the importance of chromium is placed by the growing child in the womb upon the mother. A newborn infant has hair chromium levels up to four times greater than that of the mother. Evidence has shown that hair content of chromium may be a good indicator of tissue chromium levels.

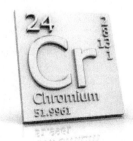

Furthermore, hair chromium levels of women who have borne children are much lower than that of women who are childless. This would seem to indicate that pregnant women do not generally consume chromium in sufficient amounts to provide for their own needs and that of their preborn children at the same time.

Yet further studies have shown that hair chromium content of a mother does not decrease after her first pregnancy. In other words, the baby sucks up her stores of chromium. This calls into question whether children after the firstborn start life with an optimum level of chromium in their bodies.

Finally, premature infants and those with evidence of growth retardation within the womb have significantly lower hair chromium content as compared to healthy infants that are born at full term. The evidence overwhelmingly supports that chromium is an important part in healthy growth for the developing child during pregnancy. In order to properly understand this concept, we need to cover some simple, basic concepts.

Conception of new life begins a process of rapid cell duplication by division (mitosis) over and over again. This requires energy ... **lots and lots of energy!** A substance named adenosine triphosphate (ATP) provides energy in human cells. ATP is the basic energy unit of the cell. If there is no ATP then there is no cell duplication. It is just that simple. That makes ATP a very simple priority for the healthy formation of life. The proper combining of glucose (sugar) and oxygen results in production of ATP. Therefore, it is of utmost importance that glucose is efficiently provided for life to flourish. Glucose is commonly referred to as blood sugar.

Most people have some familiarity with a connection between blood sugar and insulin. It is not very commonly known just what that connection is or how it works. Most people also very commonly know that the pancreas produces insulin. However, it is not very commonly known exactly what it is that insulin does.

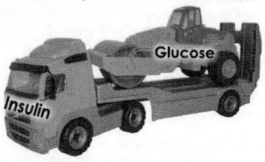

Insulin is a "transport mechanism." It is like a truck that transports glucose to cells throughout the body. Insulin delivers glucose to a cell destination. At the cell there is an insulin receptor site. An insulin receptor site is comparable to a loading dock. This is where the glucose is unloaded and passed into the cell for production of ATP (energy). If a truck pulled up with its load to a loading dock and nobody was there then how would the truck get unloaded?

Schwarz Mertz & GTF

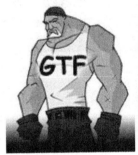

A compound named **Glucose Tolerance Factor** (GTF) is comparable to a dock worker. GTF "dock workers" move the glucose "load" from the insulin "truck" to the insulin receptor site "loading dock" and into the cell for onsite production of ATP (energy). The complete makeup of GTF is still a mystery more than half a century after being discovered by Dr. Klaus Schwarz, M.D. in 1959 with his assistant Dr. Walter Mertz, M.D. at the National Institutes of Health. However, the mineral element chromium was identified as the largest portion of the GTF compound.

GTF chromium is a shining knight whose protective armor has never been uncovered. All the king's horses and all the king's men have not been able to get GTF chromium all the way apart, so they can't figure a way to construct it or put it together again.

If there are not enough dock workers (GTF chromium) at the loading dock (insulin receptor site) then work slows and becomes inefficient. The absence of GTF chromium "dock workers" may result in a traffic jam of insulin "trucks" filled with glucose "blood sugar". This results in what is called "high blood sugar" of which the chronic state is called diabetes. If you want to keep up good, quality production in the formation of new life then plenty of GTF chromium "dockworkers" are required.

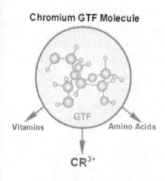

Chromium GTF Molecule

Vitamins — GTF — Amino Acids

CR^{3+}

More than half a century ago Dr. Klaus Schwarz and Dr. Walter Mertz came to the National Institutes of Health as visiting scientists from Germany. In only a few years time Dr. Schwarz had established that the mineral selenium was an essential nutrient. Previously it had been considered a poisonous element. Shortly thereafter Schwarz and Mertz working together isolated a substance found in food that corrected abnormal sugar metabolism.

Schwarz and Mertz gave this substance the name of Glucose Tolerance Factor, now commonly known as "GTF." This name was given because it restored normal sugar metabolism when diabetic tendencies were present. The GTF molecule was found to consist primarily of the mineral chromium. Schwarz and Mertz soon discovered that simple chromium salts had almost no effect at all in the human body. It was only chromium incorporated in food that had a dramatic effect.

One year after the GTF discovery had been made it was barely known at all. It was in that year (1960) that Dr. Henry A. Schroeder, a professor of medical physiology at Dartmouth University, began to conduct experiments with three different minerals. One of the three was **chromium**. Dr. Schroeder discovered that low chromium levels resulted in high blood sugar levels. Schroeder discovered that blood sugar levels decreased in accordance with how much chromium levels were increased. Schroeder also discovered that chromium deficiency is **the primary cause** of heart disease. Schroeder was noted with awards from the American Heart Association. His discovery of the chromium connection to heart disease was ignored in spite of his credentials.

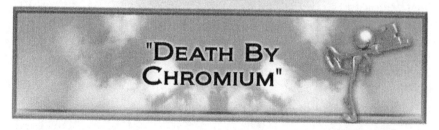

"DEATH BY CHROMIUM"

"*Death by chromium*" is something that you will **never** see on a coroner's report. Why? Because the element chromium by itself has **never** been found to be toxic at any level of usage. It has been tested safe at levels up to 10,000 micrograms.

Common, simple salts of chromium such as chromium chloride are only absorbed at a level of less than 0.5% (that is less than ½ of 1%). They are virtually nonexistent, in other words. The "experts" have told us for decades that chromium supplements are very difficult for the body to metabolize because of this. It has become a mantra against chromium supplementation. However, between 10% and 25% of chromium in food is absorbed. That is more than 20 to 50 times greater than that of chromium chloride.

Let's put that in perspective. If you consume only 50 pounds of refined, white sugar each year then your consumption is less than that of the average American. (American sugar consumption has exceeded more than 100 pounds annually for decades.) 50 pounds of refined, white sugar has had 7500 micrograms of food chromium **removed**, which amounts to more than 20 micrograms of food chromium every day. Replacing that with chromium chloride would require 400 to 1,000 micrograms every day. If you consume more than 50 pounds of refined, white sugar annually that amount goes up. The difference is much more dramatic when you bring the same comparison to refined, white flour versus whole-wheat flour.

As we've mentioned many times already, due to the lack of selenium and many other reasons, the standard American diet is "SAD." But now we can unequivocally state that the standard American diet is doubly damning because it is exceedingly deficient in the mineral chromium. The stripping of chromium from foods that normally contain the mineral then induces the body to give up its own storage levels of the element. This "SAD" status is one that leaves people in a literal world of hurt.

Like selenium, refining of flour and sugar strips almost all of the chromium from food sources. Flour (grains) and sugar cane are far and away the highest naturally occurring chromium foods commonly consumed, but the refining process renders them virtually devoid of this precious element. It should be of significant interest that sugar requires chromium to be processed fully and efficiently in the human body, and as mentioned above, sugar cane is one of the highest sources of chromium. However, when sugar cane is refined into white sugar, it loses more than 95% of its chromium. So, much like selenium, it is important to supplement with chromium, since the food supply is broken.

Both of our families take "Innate Response" chromium, which can also be found at www.choosetobehealthy.com. Much of this section on selenium was excerpted (with permission) from Chris Barr's booklet about this crucial trace element, where he reveals that "*chromium is the single most important nutrient discovered to date, yet, very few know very much at all about it -- and what little is commonly 'known' is not even correct.*"

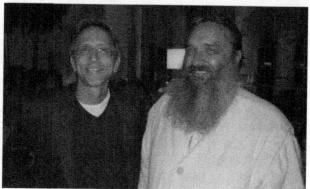

RSB with Chris Barr at the 2013 Health Freedom Expo in Chicago

"BARE BONE BASICS" ELUDE MEDICAL BONEHEADS

Diabetic women have more than twice the rate of hip fracture compared to non-diabetic women. This finding was disclosed in a recent issue of the medical journal *Diabetic Care* based upon a study exceeding 20 years duration with more than 100,000 women.

The reason this occurs was noted as "not entirely clear" to the medical researchers that conducted the study. A more accurate notation would have been "without a clue." Thinking medically rather than nutritionally often leaves researchers clueless.

Here's a clue ... or two or three ...

Let's recap what we previously mentioned. Recent figures indicate that the standard American dietary (SAD) choices consist of 20%

refined, white flour. Whole grain prior to being refined down to white flour is rich in the mineral chromium. Processing removes 91% of that chromium.

Chromium is an essential nutrient for life specifically for blood sugar metabolism. Consuming 20% of your diet from food with 91% of the chromium removed is a menu to impede blood sugar metabolism. Diabetes is a disorder of impeded blood sugar metabolism.

As Paul Harvey used to say, here is "the rest of the story." Prior to being refined, whole grain is also rich in the mineral **silicon**. Processing removes 95% of that silicon. Silicon serves a great many functions in the body. One of the most dramatic areas of need for silicon is bone strength. Consuming 20% of your diet from food with 95% of the silicon removed is a menu to diminish bone strength.

Prior to being refined, whole grain is also rich in the mineral **magnesium**. Processing removes 75% of that magnesium. Magnesium also serves a great many functions in the body. One important need for magnesium is bone strength. Consuming 20% of your diet from food with 75% of the magnesium removed is a menu to diminish bone strength. Hip fracture is a result of diminished bone strength.

The same "SAD" choices that lead to 20% of food intake from refined, white flour dramatically reduces both the anti-diabetic mineral chromium, and the bone strengthening minerals silicon and magnesium. Decades of "SAD" choices create a gross deficiency of minerals. Changing your choices may stop the deficit from increasing but will not fill in the gaping holes you have dug for yourself. Supplementation becomes an issue at this juncture. The quality of your supplementation will significantly impact your quality of life.

Chromium and silicon supplements are only efficient in 100% whole food or vegetal forms. Magnesium is most efficient in a 100% whole food form though it may still have some effectiveness in other form. Supplementation with the minerals silicon and magnesium in vegetal or 100% whole food forms is a winning strategy for bone health of diabetics and non-diabetics alike.

Much of this section was excerpted (with permission) from Chris Barr's website, www.NotaDoc.org. **NotAD℞c.org**
Our name IS our disclaimer

Have a heart, not a heart surgeon!

Now that you have had a crash course in the 3 most important mineral deficiencies affecting millions of people who have grown up under a medical monopoly, here's a bonus tip for great cardiovascular health: We cannot overstate the importance of all three (Chromium, Selenium, Silicon) working together regarding the prevention of heart disease!

1. Chromium feeds/nourishes and delivers the energy needed by the most active muscle in your body!
2. Selenium protects from the oxidative damage that would normally lead to coronary occlusion (blockage) and;
3. Silicon is critical for structural repair and integrity (strength and elasticity).

VITAMIN D - "NATURE'S GIFT"

Ultraviolet light from the sun comes in two main wavelengths – ultraviolet A ("UVA") and ultraviolet B ("UVB"). Think of UVA as the "bad guy" and UVB as "the good guy," since UVA penetrates the skin more deeply and causes more free radical damage, whereas UVB helps your skin produce vitamin D. Technically speaking, vitamin D is not really a vitamin, per se, but is more appropriately classified as a "prohormone."

Regardless, vitamin D has been shown to be crucial in preventing cancer. The mechanisms by which vitamin D reduces the risk of cancer are fairly well understood. They include enhancing calcium absorption, inducing cell differentiation, increasing apoptosis (programmed cell death), reducing metastasis and proliferation, and reducing angiogenesis (formation of new blood vessels).

So, where do I buy the best vitamin D supplement? The truth be told, most vitamin D supplements are virtually worthless. Here's why: The vitamin D in milk and in most vitamin supplements is vitamin D2 and is synthetic. Vitamin D2 is also called "ergocalciferol." It is **not** the form of vitamin D that you need to prevent cancer and degenerative diseases. In actuality, the form of vitamin D which you need is vitamin D3 (aka "cholecalciferol") and is produced from the UVB rays in sunlight. That's why I frequently refer to sunshine as the "*most affordable cancer-fighting nutrient in the world.*" Think about it, you can get a lifetime supply for **free**!

Don't fall for the "sunscreen myth." Despite what we hear from the Medical Mafia, sunlight is actually good for you (especially the UVB rays), and sunscreens filter out UVB! The main chemical used in sunscreens to filter out UVB is octyl methoxycinnamate (aka "OMC") which has been shown to kill mouse cells even at low doses. Plus, it was also shown to be particularly toxic when exposed to sunshine. And guess what? OMC is present in **90%** of sunscreen brands! The most popular brands of sunscreens also contain other toxic chemicals (such as dioxybenzone and oxybenzone) that are absorbed through the skin where they enter the bloodstream, generate free radicals, wreak havoc on the immune system, damage the liver and the heart, and even promote systemic cancer.

The time required in the sun is probably 15 to 30 minutes per day. Your needs may differ depending upon your unique skin pigmentation. The darker your skin, the more sun exposure you need to produce adequate Vitamin D levels sufficient for your needs. The optimal time for UVB production of vitamin D is around the middle of the day when the ratio of UVB to UVA is highest and the required exposure times are shortest. However, this works only when the sun is elevated high enough. During winter months, it is oftentimes impossible to produce any vitamin D from sunlight, depending upon how far north you live.

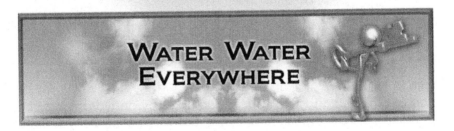

WATER WATER EVERYWHERE

Water is probably the **most important** topic. Without food, most humans will die in a month. Without water, we're dead in less than ten days. Water makes up over 70% of the body, around 90% of the blood, and about 85% of the brain.

We cannot go one day without water being a part of our life. We drink it, cook with it, bathe in it, swim in it, give thanks for it when it rains and play in it when it snows. Whether a layman or a scientist, there is no doubt that water is an integral part of each of us and the world we live in.

However, as common as it is, we still don't understand all of the amazing characteristics, capabilities and properties of water. How is it possible for the chemistry and structure of water to change 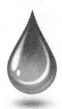 when music is played? How does placing a glass of water on a magnet change the pH? Why does ice float when other substances become heavier when turned to a solid? Scientists are baffled at some of the properties of water. Our body is 70-80% water. Beyond hydration, what is the true purpose of water in our body? Most of us just think of water as what we drink when we are thirsty or what we use to wash our hands.

Consider the following:

- ➢ 78% of all Americans are chronically dehydrated.
- ➢ The thirst mechanism is mistaken for hunger pangs in 37% of Americans.
- ➢ Mild dehydration will slow down metabolism as much as 3%.
- ➢ Drinking 8oz. of water stops midnight hunger.
- ➢ Lack of water is the leading cause of fatigue.
- ➢ A 2% reduction of water in the body can cause short-term memory loss and difficulty with basic math.
- ➢ Drinking 8 to12 glasses of water a day can reduce back and joint pain.
- ➢ Drinking 5 glasses of water daily decreases the risk of breast cancer by 79% and bladder cancer by 50%.

Visit www.RobertsWater.com to hear an interview RSB conducted with Dr. Batmanghelidj about *Your Body's Many Cries For Water*. If you are thirsty, it means your cells are already dehydrated. A dry mouth should be regarded as the last outward sign of dehydration. That's because thirst does not develop until body fluids are depleted well below levels required for optimal functioning. Some statistics show that as much as 90% of us are walking around in a chronic state of dehydration. One way to tell if you're dehydrated is to check the color of the urine. If it's dark all the time, you're probably dehydrated.

The majority of people simply don't drink enough water. For this reason a vast majority of the U.S. populace is chronically dehydrated. The definition of dehydration is when the body loses more fluid than it takes in. So, why don't people drink enough water when they know how important it is? Taste is a huge factor. Quality is another major deterrent. People are concerned with the quality of water they drink and rightly so. The news reports our water sources are being polluted, contaminated and depleted. A study of 27 water municipalities found lead, arsenic, class 3 narcotics and other harmful pollutants present in drinking water.

An alarming study released in January 2014 showed that there were 24,500 chemicals in bottled water that are known to cause cancer, gynecological issues, and 90% reduction in estrogenic receptor activity and 60% androgenic receptor activity. http://www.echowaterionizer.com/wp-content/uploads/24500-chemicals-found-in-top-18-brands-of-bottled-water.pdf Bottled water companies market bottled water as more healthy and clean. Who could have ever imagined people would pay $2-$6 for a bottle of water that actually has more contaminants than many municipal water systems?

As previously stated tap water can have any number of impurities despite the "purification" methods used by city municipalities. What most people don't know is typically the water we drink, including tap water, bottled water and filtered water carries a positive electrical charge, which is oxidative and not helpful to the body. Ionized water is a better choice than any other type of water because of taste, texture, cleanliness, cost per gallon, ease of use and most importantly, its powerful antioxidant properties due to its negative charge. Knowing how much healthier ionized water is will be the first step in changing your life for the better. But with so many water ionizers on the market, you may ask "How do I know which is the best one for me?"

What about the idea of micro clustering of water molecules? In the 1980s this idea seemed to be verified by Nuclear Magnetic Resonance (NMR) studies, which showed that ionized water had a lower than normal bandwidth. However, many recent and more accurate studies have shown that the NMR bandwidth is a function of pH not water cluster size. Additional research has completely refuted the concept of micro clustering. In 1995, some researchers suggested that atomic hydrogen (i.e. one hydrogen atom), also called "active hydrogen", was somehow stabilized and was responsible for the miraculous benefits of ionized water. However, atomic hydrogen is an unstable short-lived free radical and has thus been rightfully dismissed. Could an actual validated form of hydrogen released from H2O by electrolysis be the answer to the mystery of the benefits of ionized water?

What is Ionized Water and How Does It Work?

Electrolysis of water has been used for decades for the production of hydrogen gas for fuel. It converts water to hydrogen gas (H_2) and hydroxide ions (OH^-) at the negative side, and oxygen gas (O_2) and hydrogen ions (H^+) at the positive side. Water ionizers have a membrane that separate

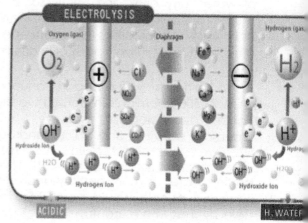

the alkaline OH^- ions from the acidic H^+ ions. The outlet from one side of the membrane gives alkaline water, which contains therapeutic dissolved hydrogen gas (H_2), and the other side of the membrane gives acidic water, containing dissolved oxygen gas (O_2).

Why is H_2 Important to the Water Ionizer User?

The H_2 molecule, unlike other antioxidants, is a selective antioxidant that *only* targets the dangerous free radicals like the hydroxyl radical (HO^*), converting them instantaneously to water. It can also prevent oxidative stress by increasing the body's own antioxidants like glutathione. It also has other beneficial cell signaling properties.

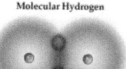

Molecular Hydrogen

Dissolved hydrogen gas or molecular hydrogen is responsible for the negative oxidation reduction potential (ORP) and the antioxidant properties of the alkaline water. The hydroxide (OH^-) ions are responsible for the alkaline pH, but they are not antioxidants themselves.

66

Finally in 2007, it was clearly shown that hydrogen gas can act as a selective antioxidant and has the therapeutic properties observed with ionized water. No one had investigated hydrogen gas before: everyone assumed it was just an inert byproduct of electrolysis - with no biological effect. If we remove hydrogen gas from ionized water the therapeutic effects are lost. When we add additional hydrogen gas to ionized water (e.g. via bubbling) the positive benefits, in many cases, are increased.

The biological effects of hydrogen gas have now been confirmed in over 600 studies and on 150 different human diseases and disease models. H_2 has been shown to be therapeutic in virtually every organ of the human body. To learn more visit www.MolecularHydrogenFoundation.com.

In 2010, after 10 years in the industry, Synergy Science, Inc. developed the premier Echo® brand of water ionizers to produce the best water ionizer in the world. They focused on producing the highest amount of H2, improved filtration, no scale buildup, attractive look, ease of use, provided installation at no charge, provided a Forever warranty, low monthly payments, and exceptional support and education. Understanding that most consumers did not want a water ionizer on top of their counter, they developed the first ionizer that could be used above counter or under sink.

The Echo® Water Ionizer has the most advanced technologies available. Unlike other water ionizers, the Echo® Water Ionizer has a patented anti-scale technology that stops scale (calcium) from attaching to the electrodes in the water cell which is inside the ionizer. Drinking Echo® Ionized Water is one of the best things you can do to improve health and wellness. You can purchase an Echo® by calling 1-800-337-7017 and speaking to our good friend, Paul Barattiero, to whom we are extremely grateful. Paul provides scientific validation and innovation in the development of reliable technologies to purify, ionize, alkalize, and release the most molecular hydrogen in water for powerful antioxidant potential and enhanced detoxification. He added much to our understanding of what this technology can do and why H_2 structured water is a **critical part** of unlocking the power to heal!

ZAP THE "BAD GUYS" WITH ZEOLITES

Zeolites are natural volcanic minerals with a unique, complex crystalline structure. Zeolites, in general, have been used for almost 1,000 years as a traditional remedy throughout Asia to promote overall health. One amazing property of zeolites is that their honeycomb framework of cavities and channels (like cages) work at the cellular level trapping heavy metals and toxins. As you know, toxins poison our air, our water, our food, and our bodies. According to the EPA, 80,000 chemicals are used commercially in the United States, and 75,000 of them are potentially hazardous to our health. The Environmental Defense Council reports that more than four billion pounds of toxic chemicals are released into the environment each year, including 72 million pounds of known carcinogens.

Zeolites are one of the few negatively charged minerals in nature. Basically, they act as magnets, attracting positively charged heavy metals and toxins, capturing them, and removing them from the body. They are an extremely effective chelating agent. Here's how: within the structure of the zeolites, there are certain "cages," inside of which are positive ions. The positive ions switch places with the heavy metals, pesticides, or herbicides, which are also positive ions, and then the cage structure of zeolites tightly binds them. One amazing quality of this "caged binding" effect is that the toxins and heavy metals are 100% excreted. In other words, they don't get "relocated" to another spot in the body, they actually get evicted!

Zeolites are effective against harsh microorganisms such as bacillus, mildew, staphylococcus, streptococcus, and fungi. They function as a broad spectrum antiviral agent, help balance pH levels in the body, reduce allergic reactions, chelate heavy metals, neutralize acids, increase oxygen levels, fend off microorganisms, and support immune system function. The main problem with zeolites is that they all "push" aluminum and lead into gastric acid, so there are other "complementary" products that **must** be used alongside of zeolites, in order to minimize their "heavy metal

68

footprint." To learn more about these products, please visit http://www.ToxinsAway.com.

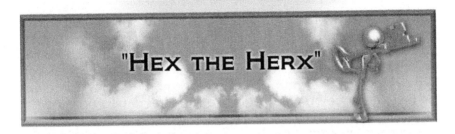

"HEX THE HERX"

People often ask me if there are any side effects to using silver hydrosol or the silver-aloe protocol for gut health recovery. Since we are not using toxic quantities of any substance in support of health recovery, side effects are not a consideration, but side benefits are. This does not mean that there are no pangs of discomfort during the healing process. Mom and grandma often tell their kids and grandkids that they might feel worse before they are better.

But why?

In homeopathy, the *"feeling worse before recovery"* is often called a healing crisis, or aggravation. In medical circles, it is typically called a Herxheimer response. It is most often seen when using antimicrobial drugs against infectious agents, especially when the die-off response in the body creates more immune debris than the body can successfully excrete in short order. Whenever there is an immune battle, even one that is successfully won, the battlefield is strewn with dead bodies that must removed in order for the terrain to fully recover. Can you imagine what the body is like when the dead microbial bodies are not removed? It's one thing to kill Candida albicans, but you better be sure that your detoxification pathways are open wide, or else you may suffer feelings of sickness, malaise, headache, bloating and more as the circulating debris remains stuck in the body. So what is the key to minimize or eliminate the potential for a Herxheimer response while on the road to recovery? The liver.

Clear the terrain. All hands on deck in support of your organs of elimination! This is why it is advisable to increase daily selenium intake while on any healing protocol that strengthens immunity. Along with selenium, NAC helps to facilitate the production of glutathione, which helps to bind the bad guys and escort them out of the body. Non-denatured whey protein is the food that increases glutathione production more than any other, also because of its high cysteine content. (www.OneWorldWhey.com)

Homeopathic drainage remedies are also a simple, yet critical metabolic support for all of the body's detoxification pathways. Whether you choose Bryonia, Chelidonium or Nux vomica for the liver, or King Bio combination formulas that stimulate the liver, kidneys, colon and lymph, these metabolic medicines can often be the difference between aggravation crises or healing ease.

Of course, all the many methods, substances and energy remedies would go for naught if you forgot the one compound that makes it all work: water! Particularly the ionized and hydrogen-enriched H_2O discussed earlier in this book. **Do I hear an ECHO?** Deep cellular hydration provides the rivers upon which all things are removed from the body.

We know that you want to be *all-better*, **yesterday**, but you can't rush healing, even though we have provided many more direct paths to healing in this book. So honor your body's needs during these challenging recovery periods. How? Get some rest! Your body is redirecting energies to complete detoxification and regeneration! When you recover by applying the information found here, your gains will not be fleeting. They will be built on a more solid foundation of healing principles that stand the test of time. Go forth! You now have the keys to **unlock the power to heal!**

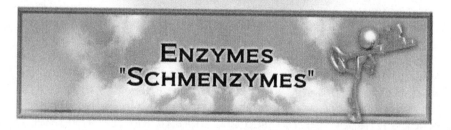

ENZYMES "SCHMENZYMES"

Many people take **enzymes** in the form of dietary supplements to replace the enzymes their bodies are lacking, or to fortify the enzymes found in their food to ensure complete digestion of each meal. If you don't digest the food, you can't absorb the nutrients. If you don't absorb the nutrients, you can't get all the fuel you need for repair, growth and learning.

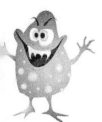

In technical terminology, enzymes are "catalysts." Just in case you were taking a nap (or staring at the pimples on your nose) during high school chemistry, a catalyst is a substance which causes a chemical reaction to take place without, itself, becoming a part of that chemical reaction.

There are several thousand different enzymes found in the human body. These enzymes can combine with coenzymes (non-protein molecules) to form nearly 100,000 various chemicals that enable us to see, hear, feel, move, digest food, and think.

Enzymes are responsible for digestion, absorption, transporting, metabolizing, and eliminating the waste of nutrients. Every organ, every tissue, and the approximate 100 trillion cells in our body depend upon enzymes.

In the body, enzymes made by **"friendly flora"** in our digestive system work synergistically with our own inherent enzymes to support optimal wellbeing and digestive health.

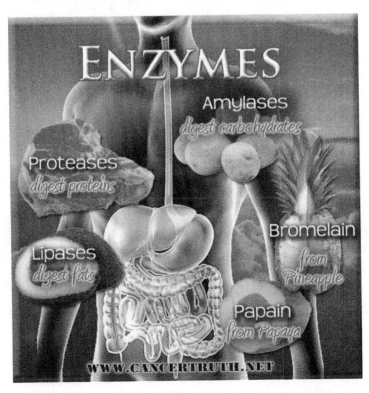

Supplementing with digestive enzymes and probiotics as a regular part of your health maintenance program provides a little insurance that you (and your family) have the tools necessary to digest everything you put in your body to get the maximum benefit, and that you are maintaining an environment in your digestive tract that will allow you to absorb all available nutrients, and continue to keep you healthy and allow you to flourish. A properly functioning intestinal tract is one of your body's main defenses against illness.

There are three major classes of enzymes: **metabolic** enzymes (enzymes which work in blood, tissues, and organs), **food** enzymes from raw food, and **digestive** enzymes. There are also three main categories of digestive enzymes: proteases (for protein digestion), amylases (for carbohydrate digestion), and lipases (for fat digestion). Remember that enzymes are just pieces of the overall digestive puzzle.

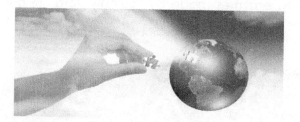

As we mentioned earlier, for enzymes to actually perform thousands of tasks, they need help from vitamins and minerals (cofactors). The enzyme and the cofactors orchestrate themselves in a complicated biochemical opus called a "complex." It is the enzyme **complex** that brings about the essential enzyme activity.

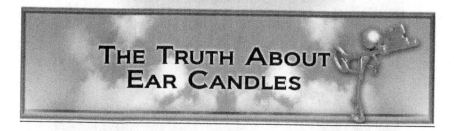

THE TRUTH ABOUT EAR CANDLES

Anyone who has suffered repeatedly with ear infections through childhood (as I did) may be a little curious about ear candles. We have used them personally and with our children to address both sinus and ear issues, but what do they actually do? Are they like a

Hoover vacuum for earwax removal? No. They interact in more subtle ways with the energy centers of the head while simultaneously impacting the terrain of the ears, nose and throat.

We are very grateful to Doc Harmony (http://harmonycone.com/harmonys-story/) for helping us to sift through the myths and get to the ear candle realities genuinely needed to clear our heads.

Do ear candles remove wax?

For a long time, people have believed this to be a truth and many ear candle companies promoted the idea because it made selling ear candles rather easy. Even though you may have a slight pulling sensation while candling, there is simply not enough suction to pull anything of consequence out of your ear canal. While it is true that there is residue at the bottom of the candle once used, it is debris from the burn, not wax from within your ear. Should a manufacturer of candles make such a claim, the FDA would demand proof of safety and efficacy for an *"unapproved new medical device."*

So what does it do? It clears the terrain on an atmospheric and energetic level. What happens when you reduce the humidity of a cave? A moist environment with sticky mud begins to dry out, allowing debris to more easily be swept, or fall out. Infectious bacteria need a fluid medium in order to reproduce. Even though an ear candle is not an anti-microbial, changing the environment makes the ear canal a less hospitable environment for the proverbial bacterial bad guys to proliferate. I typically recommend homeopathic medicine, particularly Capsicum 12x (especially for infants) or a combination homeopathic earache formula, along with flooding the ear canal with bioactive silver hydrosol. The perfect follow up? Ear candles. Simon says, "Dry up!"

What of the more energetic, perhaps esoteric benefits of ear candling? The biggest benefit, especially for adults, may in fact be stress reduction. Doc Harmony, PhD, revealed something entirely new about the benefits of ear candling recently. How? By focusing on the shift of the body to a parasympathetic state, allowing for an experience of a sense of wellbeing in times of pressure, tension, and stress. It seems so simple, but the 10-20 minute process itself often results in a meditative state via this parasympathetic expression. How valuable is relaxation? The last time we checked, stress ranked #1 on most lists when considering disease manifestation and mortality. The greatest reward may be derived from this esoteric, yet practical experience while the ear candle

73

slowly burns. Should this be the focus of candling, much like you would direct your attention on a prayerful, meditative or yoga exercise? Sounds good to us!

Another consideration is the vortex motion evident in the smoke coming from the candle. The spiral movement of the smoke indicates a very real shift of energy. The vortexing of water is what alters its energy during the production of homeopathic medicines. When you finish an ear candling session and describe a clearer head, sinus congestion notwithstanding, you experience an opening or clearing of what some call chakra energy. This may have something to do with proximity to the auricular acupuncture/acupressure points. In either case, clarity is good.

When can I use ear candles?

This could be a "Moment of Duh." Any symptoms that are proximal to conditions of the ears, nose and throat call for candling. Clearing the terrain of the ear canal also benefits the throat and sinuses because of the direct pathways linking them all. Cold, allergies, congestion, sore throat? Obviously. In a more general sense, candle when you are feeling internal stress, whether you are overwhelmed, under pressure, or feeling under the weather. These internal stresses can be emotional, spiritual, or mental and they may manifest as a headache or migraine. You can use ear candles to help the body return to homeostasis. When you ear candle, you will likely feel stress fade away. This is also known to be a return to a parasympathetic state. We have used ear candles when we experience a Type A day, whether or not there was an accompanying ear infection, sinus infection or migraine.

Are there any times or conditions for which ear candling may be contraindicated? Please consult with an ear, nose and throat specialist should you have a perforated eardrum or any open wounds in the ear canal before using an ear candle.

Could ear candling be considered part of a synergistic wellbeing protocol? Absolutely. Ear Candles, when used properly, gives the user the opportunity to shift to a parasympathetic (rest and digest) state. There is a small percentage of people that do not find the practice of ear candling relaxing as they carry a fear of a burning candle being too close to their head. We utilize and recommend Harmony Cone Ear Candles for their quality (non-GMO certified organic cotton, wax and a patented system to prevent the candle from burning below a safe level).

Is there any device that validates the science behind the ear candle?

The effects of heat and pressure fluctuation are measurable parameters. Dr. Rüdiger Schellenberg utilized a quantitative image-generating electroencephalogram to record stressed out patients before and after ear candling. In medical science, the qEEG reveals a Brain Map representation and is well known as a method to objectively measure the status of cerebral performance. Any change in the functional state of a human being will equally cause changes in the image of brain waves. See more here: http://neurodevelopmentcenter.com/neurofeedback-2/qeeg/
The FDA has approved this type of technology to assist in the diagnosis of ADHD in children and adolescents: http://qeegsupport.com/fda-approval-of-eeg-aid-for-adhd/

What did Dr. Schellenberg and the qEEG find? Beyond self-recognition of stress reduction during candling sessions, the qEEG confirmed a significant increase mainly in the occipital alpha performance upon the application of the ear candle. This increase could be measured in all the patients, as well as in the functional states, ie: eyes open. There was a more pronounced change when the eyes were closed, similar to meditation. The increase in the alpha performance is released by the practice of ear candling.

Measured in another way, the results reveal:
- A decrease of the cardiac rate and respiration frequency
- Peripheral blood vessel tone is equally reduced
- Peripheral circulation is increased.

The processes measured in the qEEG reflect a central relaxation mechanism, which also induces the change in the vegetative excitation level, which in turn is related to a relaxation of the peripheral blood vessels. This is how the circulation of the peripheral blood is improved ... **MORE OPEN, LESS PRESSURE, LESS STRESS, MORE FLOW.** These are measurable and reproducible physiological realities.

What is the History of Ear Candling?

According to Doc Harmony, most of what we know comes from oral traditions and stories related during many years of travel the world over, particularly speaking with healers and laypersons who have used ear candles for many years. There are many accounts from Europe and Central America, often concerning experiences of the grandmothers or elders, taking either cheese cloth, butcher paper or actually melting down a candle on cotton cloth and rolling up a candle to insert into the ear.

Other stories that you may have come across being shared on the internet came from channelings held in Sedona, Arizona in 1991, when Eleanor Bucci channeled:

> *Ear coning can be understood as an ancient healing modality - Atlantean, Mayan, Egyptian, Tibetan - which has, as many other healing practices, periodically spent time in "hiding". It was originally used in conjunction with initiation practices for spiritual leaders in order to strengthen their positions as bearers of great truths and as beacons of light in the darkness ... she channels candlings performed in the temples for spiritual purposes which would then affect the physical levels.*

We'll leave it to you to determine whether any of those claims are valid, but we would like to dispel the myth that ear candles come from the Hopi Tribe. They do not. A German company, Biosun, has used the Hopi name even though the Hopi tribe has denied the existence of ear candles in their tribe. A picture used by Biosun for marketing purposes purports to represent ear candles being used by the tribe, but actually shows a father giving prayer sticks to his son.

Doc Harmony was taught by Dr. Berryhill in 1992 when her son, Christopher was plagued for 6 months with ear infections. Dr. Berryhill, a Naturopath in Decatur, Georgia was trained at the Royal Homeopathic Hospital in England, with Dr. Trevor and Dr. Chapel about the practice of ear candling in the late 1960's. Unfortunately, this practice is no longer performed. There is information from the Native American Muscogee tribe of ear candles being formed with rolled up corn husks for use in children. Some stories from Poland indicate that candles were made there that resembled pencils. In Mexico, they have historically used rolled up newspaper! In Costa Rica, they call ear candles 'cartuchas'. A number of lay healers in America reported learning about ear candling directly from Dr. Christopher in the late 1950's.

What is the recent history of ear candling and the FDA?

On February 17, 2010, the FDA issued Warning Letters to 15 different companies: King Cone International; Indian Mountain Center; Bobalee Originals Manufacturing; International Ear Candle, LLC;

76

Home Remedies Solutions; Harmony Cone; A..J.'s Candles Inc; Wholistic Health Solutions; Wally's Natural Products Inc.; Body Tools; Health, Wealth, & Happiness; White Egret, Inc.; Brennan & McCoy; Amasha; Unisource; and Herbs, Heirlooms and Homebrew. Only three of these companies are still in business: White Egret, Wally's Natural and Harmony.

Here's the shocker reported nowhere else in the mainstream media except The Robert Scott Bell Show on Natural News Radio: **THE EXACT SAME DAY THE FDA SENT WARNING LETTERS TO 15 EAR CANDLE MANUFACTURES, THEY APPROVED THE NEW VACCINE: PREVNAR 13** -- *"With unprecedented coincidence the FDA has launched an all out war on ear candle manufactures in an effort to kill the industry the same week it approves the controversial Prevnar 13 vaccine."* http://www.fda.gov/downloads/BiologicsBloodVaccines/Vaccines/ApprovedProducts/UCM206264.pdf

According to news reports, Prevnar (7 valent pneumococcal conjugate vaccine [7vPnC]) has been shown to be effective against ear infections in children. Prevnar 13 is a new vaccine that is similar to Prevnar. It is expected that the effectiveness of Prevnar 13 against ear infections in children will be similar to that observed following Prevnar. Pfizer has committed to conduct a postmarketing study of the impact of Prevnar 13 in reducing ear infections among children. https://clinicaltrials.gov/show/NCT01199016

"Ear candle manufacturers were dumbfounded as to the FDA's forceful measures until the discovery of the FDA's timely approval of the trademarked drug PREVNAR. Prevnar is used to curb pneumonia and ear infection. However, MSNBC has reported that while the original Prevnar has aided in 34% of children using the drug, it also promoted new superbugs that caused more penicillin resistant ear infections. Side effects of Prevnar 13 include; bronchitis, asthma, influenza, viral syndrome, colitis, and congestive heart failure just to name a few." http://www.msnbc.msn.com/id/20825107/

Once again, the FDA shows us that it's really all about the money: The European Commission's approval for expanded Prevnar use has opened up a big market for Pfizer and will aid its growth in 2014 and beyond. With no significant competition in the market, the Prevnar franchise has the potential to make up for the company's revenue losses due to expiration of several patents. Prevnar is currently Pfizer's second biggest brand in terms of sales after Lyrica and could well become the biggest brand in the next couple of years. Expect the franchise's sales to increase from $3.97 billion in

2013 to $5.1 billion by the end of our forecast period. http://www.trefis.com/stock/pfe/articles/231202/recent-trials-could-help-pfizer-solidify-its-dominance-in-pneumococcal-vaccine-market/2014-03-20

Don't tell the FDA, but Prevnar vaccines comes with serious Adverse Events (http://www.flu-treatments.com/prevnar-vaccine.html):

- 558 deaths
- 555 life threatening conditions
- 238 permanent disabilities
- 2,584 hospitalizations
- 101 prolonged hospitalizations
- 8,166 emergency room cases and
- 16,155 "not serious"

How many babies have Ear Candles killed? NONE.

There were approximately 5 million ear candles sold per year in the US with only 3 reports of injury in 20 years and no litigation as a result of injury being brought upon a manufacturer dating as far back as 20 years.

Adverse Events Reports (AERs) for ear candles are both rare and questionable as substantiating evidence. Notably, HCEC has had no AER's. Of over approximately 20,000,000 ear candles that have been sold, there have been only four (4) substantive AERs—where there may have been a nexus between the adverse event and the ear candle worthy of investigation. Assuming that these alleged injuries actually occurred, and that the harm or injury is shown to be attributable to ear candle uses, which has not yet been determined, this presents an injury rate ratio of only .00000002.

None of the AER's have ever been investigated or followed up. Nor has there been a claim made against the manufacturer related to the AER.

Safety and Efficacy?   Here's how you manufacture a properly made ear candle:

There are several important criteria: The cotton, wax, a burn line label and, most importantly, your safety tip/filter. Why do we use Harmony Cone? They use the highest quality ingredients possible and they are the only company in the world to use a US patented safety tip. Doc Harmony's husband, Kevin designed and created a safety device that is inserted into each and every single ear candle that is handcrafted under the Doc Harmony/Harmony Cone name.

The tip functions in two ways:
1. If a user does not adhere to the instructions and goes below the burn line label, the safety tip prevents anything from dripping backwards into the candle. The burn line label is strategically placed on the ear candle to allow a sufficient amount of room for any residue to fall without any risk to the user.
2. The US patented safety tip allows the ear candle to burn cleaner which is fantastic as it creates a safer experience.

Harmony Cone is the only company in the world that uses Certified Organic Cotton. Considering that 96% of all cotton in the United States is now genetically modified, that is a real commitment to high environmental standards. Who would want GMO smoke flooding his ear canal, not to mention the pesticide residue?
http://www.vox.com/2014/8/12/5995087/genetically-modified-crops-rise-charts

What about the wax? It should be a high quality food grade wax, similar to what is used in chocolate, makeup and on apples, with a very high molten point and very low oil content. This is very important for the safety of the user and more than double the cost of cheap paraffin. Doc Harmony is doing it right!

The FDA does not want you to have access to ear candles!

During their meeting with the FDA, Doc Harmony and Harmony Cone (HC) were told very directly that FDA would never approve ear candles. It did not matter that they were safe and millions of health conscious Americans like to use them. HC decided to sue the FDA rather than buckle under the threat of tyranny. They created the Holistic Candler's Association and went to the Courts for a resolution. Would you stand idle and allow the government to limit your health choices?

Does the US government care about the American worker? The loss of US ear candle makers would affect 150,000 individuals and jobs. Ironically, ear candle abolition would result in a loss of $1,000,000 in taxes. It's just big government driving natural wellness companies out of business, reducing American's choices to use natural remedies, and ultimately increasing dependence on powerful drug and vaccine manufacturers.

Where can I get more information about ear candles?

The website www.earcandling.info is full of accurate and researched information. It provides details about a variety of ear candles and shares the truth about ear candling, at the same time dispelling the many (monumental) myths. You can learn more about the ear candles that RSB and TMB use at http://www.harmonycone.com. Or call (877) 570-4484.

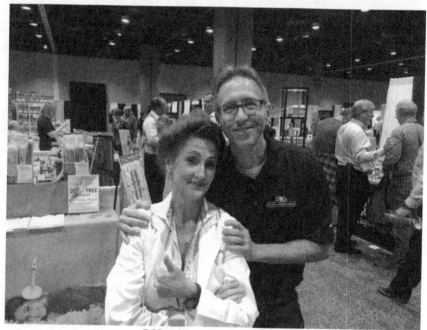

RSB with Doc Hamony

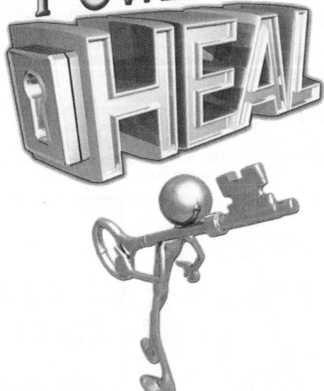

UNLOCK THE POWER TO HEAL

SECTION IV
Silver Aloe Protocol

"SILVER HYDROSOL" STOPS DOWNWARD SPIRAL OF GUT DYSBIOSIS

We live in a sea of potential enemies threatening our gastrointestinal micro flora. As mentioned above, we carry both beneficial and potentially pathogenic bacteria in our gut, but it is the **balance** that is imperative for good health. When the "bad guys" multiply due to poor diet, antibiotics, chlorinated water, food poisoning or medical drugs, this is called "dysbiosis." It is the result of polluting a pristine environment.

If health is your goal, then reversing this situation becomes imperative. Dysbiosis contributes to more serious conditions including Crohn's disease, Diverticulitis, colitis, leaky gut and irritable bowel syndrome (IBS). Chronic gut inflammation can also lead to malabsorption, metabolic shifts and obesity.

One of the really interesting new outcomes of research on **silver hydrosol** is its ability to benefit gastrointestinal health. Silver can be delivered internally to the gastrointestinal tract and offer important assistance for genuine recovery of tissue integrity. In fact, silver is essential for much more than its extraordinary antimicrobial activity. Its anti-inflammatory and tissue-regenerative properties are equally, if not more important, for recovery from chronic intestinal diseases.

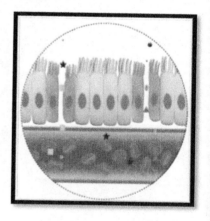

Although a number of companies use the term "silver hydrosol" for marketing purposes, there are very strict scientific criteria to determine whether a colloidal silver is, in fact, a hydrosol or not.

Are you ready for this? Technically, a silver hydrosol is an inorganic suspension of very pure (99.999%), three-dimensional, homonuclear or elemental silver nanoparticulates ≤ 10 nanometers

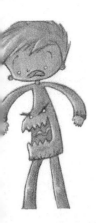

(nm) in size as the dispersed phase, stabilized by water as the continuous phase.

Particle size is a critical criterion of definition as this relates directly to inherent properties, changes in extensive properties, stability and efficiency (surface area availability). It has a CAS Registration Number (CASRN) assigned by the Chemical Abstracts Service distinct from elemental, generic colloidal and ionic silver. Demand photographic proof via electron microscopy if you are unsure if a manufacturer's claims are substantiated.

THE ROAD TO COLOSTOMY BAGS IS PAVED WITH ANTIBIOTICS & PREDNISONE

Bacterial imbalances and *Candida* overgrowth in the gut (dysbiosis) most acutely affect the epithelial tissue, including the villi. The intestinal villi are tiny, finger-like projections in the wall of the **small intestine** and have additional extensions called microvilli that protrude from **epithelial cells** lining the villi.

What do they do? As related generically (but accurately) by Wikipedia, "*They increase the absorptive area and the surface area of the intestinal wall. It is important that the food is absorbed at a considerably fast rate so as to allow more sustenance to be absorbed. If the process is too slow, the concentration of the nutrients in the blood vessels and the food will be equal, thus, diffusion will not occur. Digested nutrients (including sugars and amino acids) pass into the villi through diffusion. Circulating blood then carries these nutrients away.*"

Gut dysbiosis and inflammation damage the villi.
What substances contribute directly and indirectly to manifesting this unpleasant situation? Antibiotics, vaccines, additives, preservatives, colorings, flavorings, pesticides, herbicides, fungicides, heavy metals (mercury), "plastifiers" (BPA), GMOs and radioactive elements, just to name more than a few. In these cases, simple probiotic replenishment and fermented foods are not sufficient because the damage is too significant.

83

The toxic, inflamed, infected and deficient terrain can no longer sustain healthy microbial life forms. How do you expect life forms that are designed to live in the Brazilian rain forest to survive in the Gobi Desert? Even the best probiotics will have a great deal of difficulty colonizing such an inhospitable terrain. We'll get to the repair protocol later.

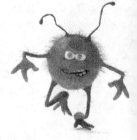

Why should you care if your villi are damaged? Nutrient absorption becomes highly impaired. Pathogenic (bad) bacteria and fungi (yeast) complicate and retard the healing process from within as they flourish in this corrupt environment. Inflammatory cytokines follow. The messengers keep sounding alerts as the imbalance does not self-resolve. The inflammation spirals out of control.

Medical doctors are trained to see this as a reason to prescribe antibiotics. When the first prescription fails, even stronger antimicrobials are prescribed. When there are no more to prescribe, the docs pull out their pads once again, this time for prednisone, a powerful steroidal drug that suppresses inflammation and immunity, while intoxicating the liver.

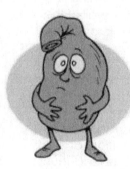

Unfortunately, for every symptom these FDA approved medicines may suppress, **additional** collateral damage is the higher price paid by your intestinal lining. Rather than balance or biosis, new levels of dysbiosis result. Many in the medical profession and millions of Americans are waking to the dangers of this standard-of-care antibiotic and steroid treatment regimen. Unfortunately, many wake up too late.

How do I define **"too late**?" Unfortunately it is when parts of your intestinal tract and colon are removed and you have to wear a colostomy bag for the rest of your life. I was confronted by just such a circumstance years ago in my homeopathic practice when a teenager came to me as a patient already wearing a colostomy bag. He had followed the medical standard-of-care to the letter after a Crohn's diagnosis. Even with all that had transpired in his young body – after all the drugs and surgery – he was still on daily doses of the antibiotic Cipro. You cannot live a long and healthy life on such a dangerous drug, with side effects including the rupturing of tendons and worse.

He was unable to form a solid stool. Even with an external pouch, chronic diarrhea is something that cannot be ignored for long. Malabsorption and dehydration are bad at any age, but hard to fathom for a 19-year-old wanting to go to medical school.

Shortly after starting a homeopathic protocol and interspersing doses of allicin-stabilized garlic and silver hydrosol, he ceased the Cipro and was able to form solid stools for the first time since undergoing medical treatment. My protocols for restoring gastrointestinal health have improved exponentially during the subsequent decade. I would like to see a time when no other teenagers are butchered by modern medicine with such needless interventions. Actually, I would like to see the same for humans of all ages!

WOULDN'T YOU RATHER HAVE SIDE "BENEFITS"?

When considering a protocol for success, you want something more natural, even intuitive, which works with your body rather than against it. Wouldn't you rather have **side benefits**, instead of side effects? Natural medicine offers more than hope. The trace element, silver, is already well known for its broad-based antimicrobial activity.

Less well understood are its remarkable anti-inflammatory and regenerative properties. Its ability to perform both functions on and in the body is actually well established, as silver is used in a wide range of medical applications from catheters and stents to antimicrobial adjuncts, antibiotics, even socks and undergarments – all for promoting protection against a sea of pathogens.

For anyone suffering from any kind of gut dysbiosis, it is important to do a thorough cleansing. In my decades of experience, silver may be the missing ingredient among all of nature's many herbal/botanical/homeopathic options.

They are preferred to antibiotics for dealing with many conditions.

Antibiotics have their important life-saving role in medicine when all else fails, but they have been overused and abused to the point of creating dangerous resistance within the microbial world. There is no resistance to the form of silver that I utilize.

Silver hydrosol, as used clinically, provides all of the antimicrobial power of drugs without the side effects. **Side effects** are actually direct effects of a drug, but are labeled as such to minimize patient resistance to pharmaceutical treatment. Please remember that abruptly stopping prescription drugs can be dangerous. The use of silver provides a nondrug option that also helps to support and modulate healthy immune activity.

Although silver can eradicate beneficial bacteria if given in large enough quantity, it certainly does not cause the collateral damage endemic to antibiotics nor does it breed microbial resistance.

HE'S BLINDED ME WITH "SILVER SCIENCE"!

Silver, as a trace mineral and normal constituent of the mammalian diet, is as aligned with the body as any natural nutrient or herbal medicine can be. After all, it is found naturally in mammalian (including human) breast milk, whole grains, medicinal mushrooms, spring water and even tap water in measurable trace amounts.[1,2]

[1]Murthy GK, Rhea U. Cadmium and Silver Content of Market Milk. (Food Protection Research; National Center for Urban and Industrial Health - US Public Health Service) Journal of Dairy Science 1968;51(4):610-613.

[2]Silver in Drinking Water; Background Document for Development of WHO Guidelines for Drinking-Water Quality. Geneva 2003. (WHO/SDE/WSH/03.04/14)

The normal physiologic pathway in humans and animals for the metabolism and elimination of ingested silver occurs in phase II liver glutathione conjugation, which leads to normal excretion as solid waste through the colon.[3]

[3]Rentz EJ. Viral Pathogens and Severe Acute Respiratory Syndrome: Oligodynamic Ag+ for Direct Immune Intervention. Journal of Nutritional and Environmental Medicine (June 2003) 13(2), 109-118.

Indeed, a strong case can be made that silver is a necessary trace element since there are natural indications that there may be receptor sites for silver in the myelin neural tissue surrounding the nerve cell, indicating benefit for the peripheral nervous system.[4,5] This is in marked contrast to heavy metals like mercury, cadmium, lead, aluminum and arsenic, which all have deleterious impact on the neuron.

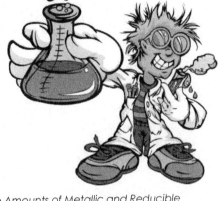

[4]Gallyas, F., "Physico-Chemical Mechanism of the Argyrophil I Reaction," Histochemistry (1982) 74:393.

[5]Gallyas, F., "Simultaneous Determination of the Amounts of Metallic and Reducible Silver in Histologic Specimens," Histochemistry, (1979) 64:77-86.

Why do we want to direct silver into the G.I. tract during recovery? We are looking to soothe the epithelial lining with its inflammation modulation activity and to clean and regenerate healthy new tissue at the site of infection and chronic injury. Silver reduces tissue inflammation.[6] I've found that silver hydrosol, followed by a quality pre- and probiotic, easily helps to eliminate all pathogenic microflora, assisting the body on its journey back to perfect balance.

[6]Wong KY, et al., "Further Evidence of the Anti-inflammatory Effects of Silver Nanoparticles." Chem Med Chem 2009, 4, p1129 – 1135.

Are you still wondering why silver is the missing component for rapid intestinal recovery? Silver accelerates tissue healing and prevents scar tissue formation.[7,8] It took me two full years to achieve recovery years before I learned of the profound healing properties of silver as manifested in silver hydrosol. I can now help others accomplish in two months or less what took me two trips around the sun to achieve when I was 26 (having started at 24). I still recommend much of what helped me over 20 years ago, but I regard the silver-aloe protocol as the most direct natural path to intestinal epithelial integrity available to everyone.

[7]Becker, RO, "Induced De-differentiation; A Possible Alternative to Embryonic Stem Cell Transplants." Neurorehabilitation 17 (2002):23-31.

[8]Jun Tian, Dr. et al. Topical Delivery of Silver Nanoparticles Promotes Wound Healing 31 Oct 2006 ChemMedChem Vol. 2 Issue 1, P. 129-136.

SILVER + ALOE = SUCCESS

When I am helping people with chronic gut issues and *Candida* overgrowth, I have them take the silver with a very good quality **Aloe vera** juice, away from meals. Ideally, the aloe should be of organic quality and free of any synthetic preservatives.

The only company I know of that ships such quality frozen is Stockton Aloe1 (http://www.aloe1.com/). Their phone number is (866) 691-0201.

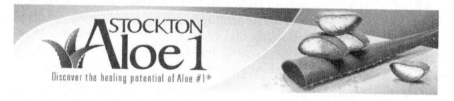

The **silver-*Aloe vera*** combination has powerful synergy, especially in carrying the active silver further along the GI tract where it is needed. I have found that silver greatly facilitates epithelial tissue and villi recovery without inflammatory side effects or creating microbial resistance. It is a great front-line defender of your health.

After intestinal recovery, a sublingual maintenance dose of silver hydrosol (one to three teaspoons per day) can be very helpful in assisting the body to guard against falling back again into bacterial disarray.

Please remember that we **only** recommend the use of bioactive silver hydrosol. Generic colloidal silvers tend to have too many compounds (salts and proteins), inactive agglomerations and inefficiently large particle sizes. What we are seeking is to maximize surface area, which only a pico- and nano-particle silver hydrosol such as Sovereign Silver® supplies.

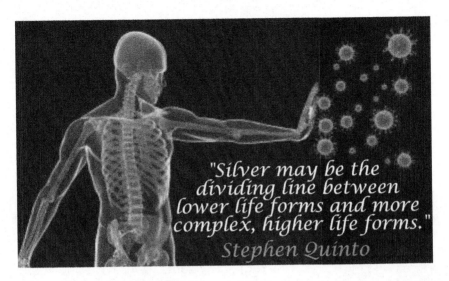

"Silver may be the dividing line between lower life forms and more complex, higher life forms."
Stephen Quinto

This, along with **Argentyn 23®** for health professionals (from the same company, Natural-Immunogenics Corp.) is the only product that we use for our families and recommend to those in need. By including it, we have not seen a more rapidly acting intestinal-health recovery protocol.

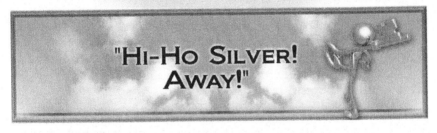

"HI-HO SILVER! AWAY!"

Adult dose: Take 1 ounce of silver with 1 ounce (or more) of aloe, swallowing directly on an empty stomach 3 times daily, followed by probiotic replenishment every evening for 1 to 2 weeks for mild dysbiosis or candida overgrowth. Those who weigh less than 120 pounds can use half the dose.

For those dealing with more serious, chronic gut inflammation, including Crohn's, IBS, leaky gut, colitis and diverticulitis, please consult with your chosen health care provider. The protocol may require 4, 6 or even 8 weeks for completion. Considering the toxic drugs and surgical butchery of allopathic medicine, this method may be much more desirable, both in economics and desired outcome. Although I do not support the indiscriminate use of antibiotics, the only class of said drugs contraindicated with the use of silver are sulfonamides (Bactrim, Septra) due to the strong affinity that silver and sulfur have for one another.

- Maintenance: 1 teaspoon daily
- Immunity-building: 3 teaspoons daily
- Chronic immune support: 5 teaspoons daily
- Gastrointestinal health: 1-2 tablespoons with aloe 3 times daily
- Acute immune support: 7 teaspoons daily

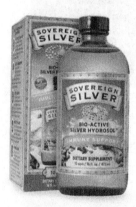

Teaspoon (5 mL/cc) doses, even when taken multiple times on a daily basis, do not disrupt normal healthy gut flora. An oral dose has to exceed 2 tablespoons (30 mL/cc) of volume, which means more than one ounce. There is a silver hydrosol preference toward pathogens because these bacteria have a negatively charged surface or negative zeta potential.

Good bacteria, such as Lactobacilliccus have a more positively charged surface. If the dose is light enough, mostly pathogenic species will be selectively killed. With a larger dose, all species are killed. So, oral dosage becomes a fine line situation. By mixing the silver with aloe gel / juice, the silver is carried farther along the lumen to kill micro-organisms lower in the gut.

MORE MAGNIFICENT REMEDIES

For those interested in the other adjunctive remedies and supplements that I utilize in order to further accelerate comprehensive recovery for those most in need, see the following:

- **1500 mg vegetal Silica** 4x (100% whole food) daily during 4-week loading phase (ALTA Health Products); reduce dose by 50% after 4 weeks; maintenance dose thereafter 500mg

3x daily ** *Purpose:* Connective tissue integrity, epithelial lining regrowth

- **Homeopathic Upper G.I. support** (King Bio 800-543-3245) as label directs ** *Purpose:* Enzymatic restoration

- **Homeopathic Lower G.I. support** (King Bio) as label directs ** *Purpose:* Probiotic restoration

- **Homeopathic Candida cleanse** (King Bio High Potency 9) as label directs ** *Purpose:* Normalize metabolic candida balance

- **Homeopathic heavy metal cleanse** (King Bio Heavy Metal Detox) as label directs ** *Purpose:* Mobilize body metabolically to excrete heavy metals including mercury

- **Non-denatured whey protein** (One World Whey 888-988-3325) as label directs ** *Purpose:* Glutathione production, detoxification, cellular repair

- **3-5 g L-glutamine** per day (or as directed on label) ** *Purpose:* Gut lining repair support

- **Essential fatty acids EPA and DHA** 3-5g daily ** *Purpose:* Inflammation reduction and modulation; cellular repair

UNLOCK THE POWER TO HEAL

SECTION V
Terrific Tips for Treating Tissue Trauma

HEALTH SOVEREIGNTY
WITH HOMEOPATHY

Obamacare is certain to hasten the demise of the medical monopoly (should it survive Constitutional challenge) by driving even more doctors out of the profession and bankrupting the system left behind. It is far past time to learn about the substances in use on the battlefields during the 19th century's War Between the States.

If you need to know surgical techniques, there are thousands of articles and authoritative texts revealing the medical methodologies in treating gunshot wounds, so I will not rehash that which you can read elsewhere. There are very few articles that address homeopathic, herbal and mineral options, especially as we approach times when government-sanctioned doctors may become scarce.

Visit any Civil War museum and you will find that both Union and Confederate soldiers carried homeopathic first aid kits. Homeopathic medicine is a 200+ year old medical system used worldwide for both acute trauma care and chronic, long term illness care.

It has been used on the battlefields throughout its history, including by the Russian General Korsakov in the war against Napoleon Bonaparte in the 19th century. Self sufficiency (or "health sovereignty" as I like to call it) in a crisis, is only made possible by knowledge of homeopathy, along with medicinal herbs and supporting minerals. These are all critical natural tools to not only have on hand – but to know how to use! I will endeavor to bring the past back to life in the care of your health should you or a loved one befall traumatic injury, particularly by gunshot.

It's time to go forward to the past...

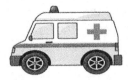 Whenever I refer to a homeopathic medicine/remedy, people are inclined to ask for what potency I recommend. The critical factor is the right remedy, **not** the right potency, so whatever is available – use it!

My preferences follow: 10x, 12x, 15x, 6c, 12c, 6x, 30x or 30c. Frequent repetitive dosing (hourly or more frequently) is necessary nearest the time of acute trauma, gradually moving to less frequent dosing as the victim improves further from crisis. The dosing schedule reduction could span from hours to days to weeks – whatever it takes. Let the body and its symptoms be your guide. If pain is present, frequent dosing is best. As pain subsides, you may space doses out further and further apart until no longer needed.

MINIMIZING BLOOD LOSS & REBUILDING PLASMA

Reducing blood loss by slowing or stopping the bleeding is **priority #1**. After applying pressure or tourniquets where needed, immediately begin dosing orally with homeopathic Bellis perennis and Phosphorus. This will accelerate bleeding cessation. Diluted **bellis** (daisy) tincture can be applied locally as well. To further promote healthy blood clotting, **Vitamin K** rich foods or supplements should also be administered. They include alfalfa, amaranth leaves, beet greens, Brussels sprouts, chard, collards, kale, mustard greens, sea kelp, spinach and turnip greens.

How do you rebuild blood plasma volume when the Red Cross is nowhere to be found? Almost lost to history, very little attention is paid to the fact that during World War II (particularly in the Pacific theatre), soldiers who had significant blood loss were given intravenous infusions of coconut water to maintain circulatory plasma volume while the red blood cells could be replenished.

Also erased from the medical history books is knowledge of French biologist and researcher Rene Quinton, who proved that you could restore life even in the case of dangerous blood loss by infusing isotonic solutions of clean sea water. In his monumental book

"L'eau de mer, milieu organique" (*"Sea Water, organic medium"*) he established scientifically the organic relationship that exists between sea water and blood plasma.

Rebuilding the blood rapidly can be assisted by increasing intake of chlorophyll, beets, alfalfa, Folate, B12, and Vitamin C – all enhancing the efficiency of iron assimilation. Homeopathic **Ferrum phosphoricum** is also very helpful for more efficient use of iron. Replenishing trace elements will greatly accelerate recovery in those who have suffered blood loss. Another means by which this is accomplished is through oral ingestion of brine from ancient sea bed mineral salts. Sea vegetation (sea weed) is another tremendous source of nutrients for rebuilding the blood.

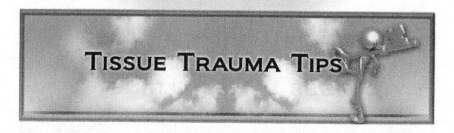

TISSUE TRAUMA TIPS

Whenever there is tissue trauma and shock, homeopathic **Arnica montana** and Arnica tincture is your best friend! The tincture can be applied topically on unbroken skin but is not for ingestion.

Should there be any bone breaks or fractures, diluted Symphytum tincture, otherwise known as Comfrey, boneset or knitbone, can be applied topically, while homeopathic **Symphytum** and **Silicea** is taken internally to speed the healing of bone tissue. Increasing dietary Silica will also greatly accelerate healthy re-growth of connective tissue, whether it is bone, cartilage, tendon, muscle, vascular or neurological.

If there is injury to the skull or brain, both Arnica and homeopathic Natrum sulfuricum are absolutely essential.

How do we prevent or eliminate infection while accelerating tissue healing with no scarring? No natural substance on planet earth does more to promote rapid healing of damage and/or infected tissue than silver.

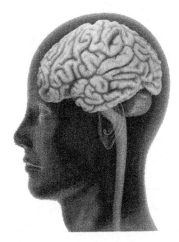

While colloidal silver can be made at home, barring end-of-world scenarios, I prefer the efficacy of silver hydrosol, which contains only the active state of silver in pharmaceutical grade purified water.

Silver reduces inflammation to damaged tissue upon contact, while simultaneously stimulating stem cell production locally for rapid restoration of tissue integrity. The process of dedifferentiation and redifferentiation of stem cells is a normal and necessary process for healthy tissue regeneration. Silver just happens to accelerate the process greatly.

It also retards and eliminates infection by disrupting bacterial and fungal membranes and can even bind with DNA so that the pathogens can no longer reproduce. If the silver particles are small enough (as they are by definition in silver hydrosol) they can bind with viral particles to prevent or reverse viral infection as well, which is critical because viral particles need damaged tissue in order to access areas of the body where the immune system is stressed.

Among the many astounding properties that are inherent to silver is the fact that it is an oxygen sponge. It can carry up to ten times its atomic weight in oxygen, the warmer it gets. This feeds copious amounts of oxygen to the white blood cells of your own immune system, enhancing the production of that which also fights infection from within: **Reactive Oxygen Species** (ROS).[1,2,3,4,5]

[1]Gan X, Liu T, Zhong J, Liu X, Li G. Effect of silver nanoparticles on the electron transfer reactivity and the catalytic activity of myoglobin. Chembiochem. 2004 Dec 3;5(12):1686-91.

[2]Samuni A, et al. On the Cytotoxicity of Vitamin C and metal ions. Eur J Biochem. 1983;99:562.

[3]Jansson, G, Harms-Ringdahl, M, "Stimulating Effects of Mercuric- and Silver Ions on the Superoxide Anion Production in Human Polymorphonuclear Leuko-cytes," Free RadicRes commun, 1993; 18(2):87-98.

[4]X. Chen*, H.J. Schluesener. Nanosilver: A nanoproduct in medical application. Toxicology Letters 176 (2008) 1–12.

[5]Park, H.J., "Silver-ion-mediated Reactive Oxygen Species generation affecting bactericidal activity." 2009 Water Research 43:1027-1032.

In addition to topical or local administration, silver hydrosol should also be taken internally, frequently (hourly) in the early stages of recovery and then less frequently as the victim is brought out of crisis. Hold the silver sublingually before swallowing, if possible, to increase absorption into the lymphatic system for maximum dispersion and immune benefit.

For those concerned about turning blue by ingesting too much silver, utilizing silver hydrosol eliminates that possibility, as it has a safety profile more like a homeopathic remedy than a silver salt.

Silver salts and other silver compounds are the forms of silver that have a difficult time being excreted from the body. See safety profile below:

Relative Toxicity by General Species of Silver
Highest ⬆ Salt solution - inorganic Salt solution - organic Salt alkali Protein complex / crystaloid Oxide Colloidal dispersion Hydrosol **Lowest** Homeopathic

Should there be tissue damage due to burns from bullets shot at close range, homeopathic **Apis** and **Cantharis** should be taken orally to reduce burn-associated pain. For nerve pain, take homeopathic **Hypericum**. Arnica should also be taken to reduce the tissue shock/trauma. Clean the area with silver hydrosol (or colloidal silver) and apply silver (soaked on sterile gauze), silver gel or silver/aloe vera combination gel as a salve and cover. Silver is also an excellent pain reducer, especially when nerve tissue is directly impacted, because the nerves cells recover rapidly in the presence of silver. This explains the normalization of sensation and function that I have seen with nerve injury and even peripheral neuropathy when dosing with silver hydrosol.

If the skin blisters, take homeopathic **Rhus tox**. If it becomes infected, first use homeopathic Arsenicum album. If the wound oozes pus, then utilize homeopathic **Hepar sulfur**. Apply silver topically throughout the healing process.

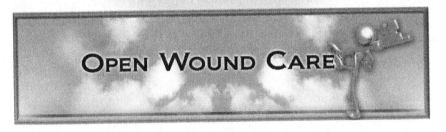

If there is poisoning due to lead bullet fragments remaining in the body, daily administration of homeopathic **Plumbum metallicum** will help the body to more efficiently deal with the burden. Increasing the trace mineral **selenium** will also assist in heavy metal removal. Use at least 200 micrograms (mcg) a day. 400 mcg may be more optimal in the presence of known heavy metal toxicity. Other substances known to bind heavy metals and remove them from the body include chlorella, spirulina, cilantro and vegetable glycerine, but be sure that they come from organic, nontoxic soils. **Far infrared heat/light saunas** are also another means by which you can accelerate metal detoxification. In the case of these saunas, you are able to release fat-soluble toxins and sweat them out through the skin, thus reducing the burden on your liver and kidneys.

Open Wound Care

In the case where wounds are very large and the skin is completely lost, silver, once again, is the top priority. 3rd degree burn care centers worldwide use a silver based medicine (**Silver sulfadiazine**) in order to accelerate skin re-growth, even when grafts are not possible. We already discussed the use of silver topically, but you can also use silver hydrosol to debride the wound as necessary as the tissue heals.

For those in southern climates, aloe vera may also be plentiful and is an ideal complement. If you do not have access to aloe, **calendula** and **echinacea** are excellent botanicals that can be used to accelerate tissue healing.

The restoration of integrity of the connective tissue (skin, bone, muscle, tendon, cartilage, nervous system, vascular system) is dependent upon adequate amounts of dietary silicon (**silica**). The highest concentrations are found in horsetail extract. I would recommend about 5000 mg per day of vegetal silica during recovery. This overlooked mineral can mean the difference of healing in weeks rather than months. The homeopathic form (**Silicea**) can be taken daily as well throughout the healing process.

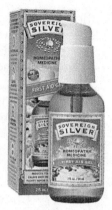

Yunnan Baiyao has been extensively used in Asia for many years and is considered a sort of miracle drug for wounds, pain, and

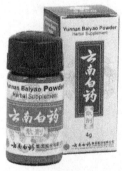

hemorrhage. It is famous for being carried in first aid kits by the Viet Cong during the Vietnam War. It has been used by Chinese soldiers for hundreds of years. It is useful for any type of open wound and any kind of surgery. It reduces recovery time for surgery by half because it mends injured blood vessels. It does not interfere with Western sedative drugs, so can be used the same day as surgery. By immediately activating blood circulation, it helps resolve bleeding, pain, and swelling. It heals oozing wounds and damaged blood vessels, while expelling pus and counteracting toxins. Cuts heal quickly with even a single application, and with a butterfly bandage it can help seal smaller wounds that might otherwise require stitches. In various clinical studies, it has shown to reduce clotting time by 33% to 55%.

PROVEN PROCEDURES TO PREVENT PAIN

I have interviewed many doctors on the subject of pain over the years on my radio show. Perhaps the most profound revelation in pain reduction came from the chief neurosurgeon for the Pittsburgh Steelers professional football team, Dr. Joseph Maroon. Rather than pharmaceutical drugs for injuries and nerve pain, he proved that EPA and DHA containing fish oils were as effective, if not more so, at reducing pain and inflammation throughout injury recovery.

There is another important botanical that is re-emerging into medicinal acceptance: **hemp**. It is rich in **Cannabidiol** (CBD) and is proving to be worth its weight in gold as a plant-based assistant in the reduction of pain and anxiety. This form of cannabis contains little or no THC, so it lacks a psychoactive component largely unnecessary in pain and anxiety reduction. Even better than that, this form of hemp oil is available in all 50 states as a dietary supplement, so it does not require an act of Congress in Washington, D.C. or any state in order for you to access it. The next section of the book will focus on this amazing plant.

Another option in the botanical family, white willow bark tincture is nature's aspirin, but is actually much safer than the synthetic aspirin approved by the FDA. **St. John's Wort** (Hypericum) is excellent for nerve pain as well, while **skullcap** (Scutellaria) is often used for reducing head-related pains.

The "granddaddy" of pain reducing botanicals is, of course, **Arnica montana** (leopard's bane), to be used topically only on unbroken skin in full strength. As an herb, it is slightly toxic to ingest, so use internally only in its homeopathic form.

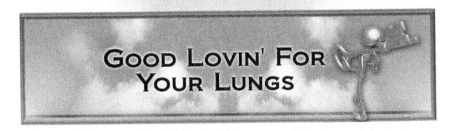

GOOD LOVIN' FOR YOUR LUNGS

Since I was the poster boy for allergies before learning of the things we have written in this book, I have extra compassion for anyone who suffers with respiratory ailments, whether it is from acute infection or chronic allergies and asthma. We've discussed the science supporting the reasons we use silver therapeutically for healing the gut, but a phone call I received many years ago from a listener of The Robert Scott Bell Show clued me into a whole new reality for recovery from serious pulmonary challenges, including multi-drug resistant pneumonias.

Joe D., a Vietnam veteran, called to explain that he had suffered with pneumonia for a full year, having gone through every antibiotic that the VA medical system could throw at him, including the most expensive, newest and most powerful ones. Nothing had worked. He related to me LIVE on the air that he had heard me discuss the use of silver hydrosol in a nebulizer for lung issues. He put one teaspoon in the nebulizer cup and breathed deeply until the cycle finished. He did this a few times over the next 24 hours and his lungs cleared completely! Pneumonia can be a very serious complication from previous infections and failed antibiotic rounds, so I am not encouraging you to ignore sound medical advice, but what will you do when their drugs fail?

Silver is not magic. It has profound properties that benefit your immune system, directly intervening in situations of microbial infections. It also down-regulates tissue inflammation when delivered to the point of foci, while simultaneously supporting healthy tissue regeneration. When there is infection within your lungs, delivering active silver at a safe level via nebulization is extraordinarily easy and not contraindicated even if you use steroid inhalers for chronic asthma. Many states require a prescription to buy a nebulizer at the pharmacy, but you can order one through online retailers without prescription.

Every home should have one for any time the kids come home with a persistent cough, or someone at the office sneezes on you. We've been using silver hydrosol in a nebulizer with our kids since they were toddlers. The bioactive silver hydrosol is already in a base of pharmaceutical grade purified water, so there is no need to dilute with additional water. One teaspoon at a time for adults, ¼ to ½ for kids. Let your body signals dictate the frequency until symptoms no longer persist. Whether it's once a day or once an hour, your body will let you know by the symptoms that are either present, improving, or absent. Please remember, this information does not take the place of qualified health care provider, nor is it intended to treat any disease. Can you handle the power to heal when it is given unto you?

Before learning of silver hydrosol, I had a number of go-to homeopathic remedies to cover most any kind of cough, asthma, and/or bronchitis; pretty much anything that affected my respiratory system. Are you ready for them?

The first remedy that follows is indicated for use no matter which of the subsequent remedies best correspond to your respiratory symptoms. Start with homeopathic **Bryonia alba**. Recommended potencies can be found in the chapter titled "Health Sovereignty with Homeopathy." Bryonia is an excellent first choice because it is a polychrest for the liver, while also being indicated for dry coughs. In Traditional Chinese Medicine, the lungs are often linked to the kidneys, which are passively downstream from the liver. Follow up remedies include **Antimonium tartaricum**, **Drosera** and **Spongia tosta**, which I jokingly refer to as Toasted Sponge Bob. For the sake of brevity, I would ask that you do more research on these remedies in the Boericke Materia Medica (or online). I do realize that fear is a big part of breathing difficulty, so you may benefit from a dose of homeopathic **Gelsemium** in those anxious moments. King Bio has complex formulations ready to go for respiratory symptoms if Latin-named single remedies overwhelm you.

One particular herb demands special attention in our discussion of respiratory health recovery, including from cases of COPD and Emphysema: **Lobelia.** While this herb can be slightly toxic when consumed to excess, used appropriately it is a miraculous medicine from the Creator to heal lung function. How best to take it? Use one dropperful of lobelia tincture diluted in a large glass of water and sip on the water over the span of a couple of hours each morning. Don't gulp it. **Sip it slowly.** Reports of recovery from the most severe of lung diseases, including the regeneration of the cilia hairs within the lung tissue are extraordinary! Although this regenerative process is not completed in one day, the reality is that there are no incurable diseases. Stay the course, stay persistent, provide the body what it needs and the substances of nature can perform miracles.

UNLOCK THE POWER TO HEAL

SECTION VI
Heavenly Hemp ...
Curative Cannabis ...
Medicinal Marijuana

MIRACLE "PLANT" OR EVIL "WEED"?

A 1938 article from *Popular Mechanics* stated that there are more than 25,000 uses for hemp ... from food, paint and fuel to clothing and construction materials. There are even hemp fibers in your Lipton® tea bags. And several cars made today contain hemp. One acre of hemp can produce as much raw fiber as 10 acres of trees. Pulping hemp for paper would produce a stronger paper that lasts incredibly long and doesn't yellow with age.

Hemp oil (derived from hemp seeds) has long been recognized as one of the most versatile and beneficial substances known to man. Hemp is considered to be a "super food" (like spirulina and chlorella) due to its high essential fatty acid content and the unique ratio of omega-3 to omega-6, specifically gamma linolenic acid (GLA). Hemp oil contains up to 5% of pure GLA, a much higher concentration than any other plant.

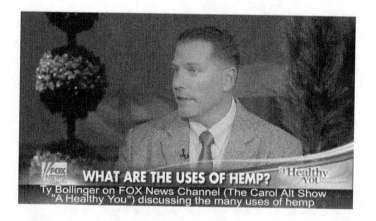

WHAT ARE THE USES OF HEMP?
Ty Bollinger on FOX News Channel (The Carol Alt Show "A Healthy You") discussing the many uses of hemp

Before we go any further, let us explain the terms "**hemp**" and "**marijuana**" and "**cannabis**."

Cannabis is scientific term that refers to the genus of the flowering plant we all know and love. It is the common glue across the three words, as both marijuana and hemp come from the cannabis plant. Three generally accepted varieties include *cannabis indica* and *cannabis sativa* and *cannabis ruderalis*.

The physical, psychoactive, and non-psychoactive effects of cannabis result from its content of **cannabinoids**, which are chemical compounds that act on human cannabinoid cell receptors that repress neurotransmitter release in the brain. These cannabinoid receptors are part of the human endocannabinoid system (ECS) which regulates relaxation, eating, sleeping, certain inflammation responses and even cognitive function. The ECS is responsible for making sure your entire body is working optimally— no small task! Two cannabinoids are preeminent in cannabis are **THC** (a psychoactive ingredient) and **CBD** (an anti-psychoactive ingredient).

Hemp is an Old English term that refers to **low THC** strains of the cannabis plant. Hemp is used for many "industrial" uses such as fuel, fiber, paper, textiles, detergents, paints, plastics, and other building materials. Hemp is also used for food, due to its highly nutritious seeds and oil. "Industrial" hemp, with its low THC content, is not a recreational or medicinal drug, nor can it effectively be used as one. The reason for the low THC content in hemp is that most THC is formed in resin glands on the buds and flowers of the female cannabis plant. Industrial hemp is not cultivated to produce buds, and therefore lacks the primary component (THC) that would get someone "high," while typically containing much higher concentrations of CBD.

"**Marijuana**" is of Spanish derivation ("*marihuana*") and has been primarily used to describe varieties of cannabis that were more commonly bred over time for medicinal and recreational purposes. The term "marijuana" was heavily pushed by US prohibitionists in the 1930s to make it sound "foreign" and "sinister" in their quest to ban the cannabis plant. Both "marijuana" and "hemp" contain the cannabinoids THC and CBD; however "marijuana" contains much **higher** concentrations of the psychoactive **THC** which produces the "high."

To be honest, we prefer to use the terms "hemp" or "cannabis" for all varietals of the cannabis plant. Using the term "marijuana" is actually acquiescing to the prohibitionists that want to ban this miracle plant ... not miracle "**drug**" ... but miracle "**plant.**"

You see, "marijuana" was one of the battle line words that marked the difference between "straights" and "stoners" ... between "Feds" and "heads."

A FEW FASCINATING FACTS

Did you know?

- Early laws in some American colonies actually required farmers to grow hemp, and they could go to jail for refusing to grow it!

- According to their diaries, many of our early presidents, including George Washington and Thomas Jefferson, grew hemp.

- The Declaration of Independence and the Constitution of the USA were both drafted on hemp paper.

- Abraham Lincoln used hemp seed oil to fuel the lamps in his home.

- Henry Ford built an experimental car body out of hemp fiber, which is 10 times stronger than steel. The first Model-T was actually built to run on hemp fuel. (*Popular Mechanics*, 1941)

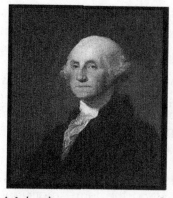 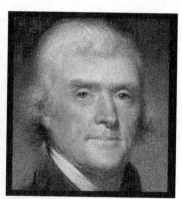

"Make the most you can of the Indian Hemp seed and sow it everywhere."
~ George Washington

"Hemp is of first necessity to the wealth and protection of the country."
~ Thomas Jefferson

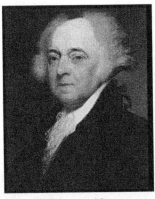 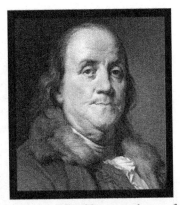

"We shall, by and by, want a world of hemp more for our own consumption." ~ John Adams

Benjamin Franklin owned one of the first paper mills that processed hemp into parchment, on which was drafted the Declaration of Independence and U.S. Constitution.

Who benefits by keeping cannabis illegal?

- The criminal underworld (with multibillion $ "businesses") thrives on its illegality

- The Drug Enforcement Administration (DEA) with a budget of upwards of $1.2 **billion** stands to lose a significant portion of its annual budget should cannabis become legal

- The prison industry benefits only with an ever-growing source of new prisoners -- 42% of all drug arrests are cannabis related. Taxpayers are spending more than $1 **billion** annually to imprison "pot" offenders (BJS report, "*Drug Use and Dependence, State and Federal Prisoners, 2004*")

- Local law enforcement receives federal grants to enforce drug laws that criminalize cannabis

- Lawyers, judges, probation officers whose jobs depend upon a steady stream of clients

- Big Pharma with its psychiatric medications, pain medications, and cancer medications

- The oil industry

- The paper/textile industry

- The agricultural chemical industry

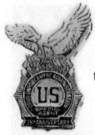

"Marijuana, in its natural form, is one of the safest therapeutically active substances known ... It would be unreasonable, arbitrary, and capricious for the DEA to continue to stand between those sufferers and the benefits of this substance."

~ *Francis L. Young, DEA Chief Administrative Law Judge, 1988*

HEMP'S HIDDEN HISTORY

For millennia, hemp has been used in medicinal teas and tonics because of its healing properties. As late as the 1930s in the USA, medicinal hemp tinctures with THC were available in most pharmacies. But in the 1940s, hemp was made illegal. But why would the US government outlaw a **plant** which has a plethora of useful applications? I'll tell you why. One main reason was that at that time, William Randolph Hearst and the Hearst Paper Manufacturing Division of Kimberly Clark owned millions of acres of timberland.

The Hearst Company, which supplied most of the paper products in the USA and also owned most of the newspapers, stood to lose billions because of the hemp industry. In 1937, Dupont patented the processes to make plastics from oil and coal. Dupont's Annual Report urged stockholders to invest in its new petrochemical division. Synthetics such as plastics, nylon, and rayon could now be made from oil. Natural hemp industrialization would have ruined over 80% of Dupont's business.

Andrew Mellon became President Hoover's Secretary of the Treasury and Dupont's primary investor. He appointed his future nephew-in-law (Harry J. Anslinger) to head the Federal Bureau of Narcotics and Dangerous Drugs. Secret meetings were held by these financial tycoons. Hemp was declared "dangerous" and a threat to their billion dollar enterprises. For their dynasties to remain intact, hemp had to go. They took an obscure Mexican slang word ("marijuana") and pushed it into the consciousness of America.

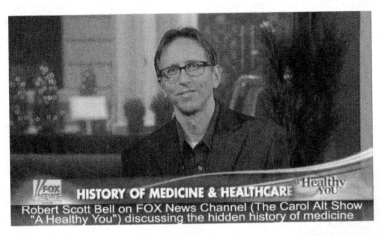

HISTORY OF MEDICINE & HEALTHCARE
Robert Scott Bell on FOX News Channel (The Carol Alt Show "A Healthy You") discussing the hidden history of medicine

A media blitz of "yellow journalism" raged in the 1920s and 1930s; Hearst's newspapers ran stories emphasizing the horrors of "marijuana." Readers were led to believe that it was responsible for car accidents, loose morality, and countless acts of violence, incurable insanity, and brutal murders. Hollywood films like "Reefer Madness" and "Marijuana: The Devil's Weed" were nothing more than blatant propaganda designed by these industrialists to create an enemy. Their purpose was to gain public support so that anti-marijuana laws could be passed. Coupled with the fact that Big Pharma didn't like the non-toxic and inexpensive medicinal applications, and you have two main reasons for "criminalizing" a glorious, medicinal plant with numerous therapeutic and industrial uses.

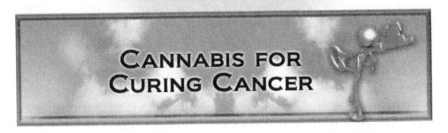

CANNABIS FOR CURING CANCER

The medical evidence for the effectiveness of THC at treating cancer and also reducing pain is overwhelming. We have known this since 1974 when the first experiment documenting hemp's anti-tumor effects took place at the Medical College of Virginia at the behest of the US government and the National Institute of Health

(NIH). The study found that THC slowed the growth of three kinds of cancer in mice (*lung and breast cancer, and a virus-induced leukemia*). Unfortunately, rather than spreading the word about the amazing medicinal properties of hemp, the DEA quickly shut down the Virginia study and all further research on the anti-cancer effects of hemp.

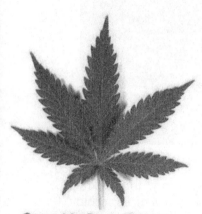

**Cannabis Cures Cancer
THIS should be the true
symbol of the fight against it.**

On March 29, 2001, the *San Antonio Current* printed a story by Raymond Cushing titled, *"Pot Shrinks Tumors – Government Knew in '74"* which detailed the suppression of news about hemp's cancer benefits, specifically relating to the 1974 Virginia study. Cushing noted in his article that it was hard to believe that the knowledge that cannabis can be used to fight cancer has been suppressed for almost thirty years and aptly concluded his article by saying: *"Millions of people have died horrible deaths and in many cases, families exhausted their savings on dangerous, toxic and expensive drugs. Now we are just beginning to realize that while marijuana has never killed anyone, marijuana prohibition has killed millions."*

In 2000, researchers in Madrid learned that the THC in hemp inhibits the spread of brain cancer through selectively inducing programmed cell death (*apoptosis*) in brain tumor cells without negatively impacting surrounding healthy cells. They were able to destroy **incurable** brain tumors in rats by injecting them with THC. But sadly, most Americans don't know anything about the Madrid discovery, since virtually no major US newspapers carried the story.

A 2007 Harvard Medical School study (published in *Science Daily*) showed that the hemp's THC decreases lung cancer tumors by 50% and significantly reduces the ability of the cancer to metastasize (spread). *"The beauty of this study is that we are showing that a substance of abuse, if used prudently, may offer a new road to therapy against lung cancer,"* said Anju Preet, Ph.D., a Harvard researcher. http://www.sciencedaily.com/releases/2007/04/070417193338.htm

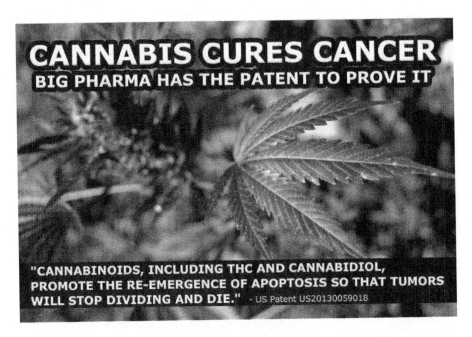

CANNABIS CURES CANCER
BIG PHARMA HAS THE PATENT TO PROVE IT

"CANNABINOIDS, INCLUDING THC AND CANNABIDIOL, PROMOTE THE RE-EMERGENCE OF APOPTOSIS SO THAT TUMORS WILL STOP DIVIDING AND DIE." - US Patent US20130059018

A recent study out of Thailand demonstrated that THC can also fight bile duct cancer, which is rare and deadly. As a matter of fact, the International Medical Verities Association is including hemp oil on its cancer protocol. Studies have also shown that hemp's cannabinoids (both **THC** and **CBD**) inhibit the proliferation of other various cancers, including:

- Breast cancer http://cancerres.aacrjournals.org/content/66/13/6615.abstract
- Colorectal cancer http://gut.bmj.com/content/54/12/1741.abstract
- Prostate cancer http://cancerres.aacrjournals.org/content/65/5/1635.abstract
- Stomach cancer http://ar.iiarjournals.org/content/33/6/2541.full.pdf
- Skin cancer http://www.jci.org/articles/view/16116
- Leukemia http://www.ncbi.nlm.nih.gov/pubmed/16908594
- Lymphoma http://onlinelibrary.wiley.com/doi/10.1002/ijc.23584/abstract
- Lung cancer http://www.nature.com/onc/journal/v27/n3/abs/1210641a.html
- Uterine cancer http://americanmarijuana.org/Guzman-Cancer.pdf
- Thyroid cancer http://www.ncbi.nlm.nih.gov/pubmed/19047095
- Pancreatic cancer http://cancerres.aacrjournals.org/content/66/13/6748.abstract
- Cervical cancer http://jnci.oxfordjournals.org/content/100/1/59.abstract
- Mouth cancer http://www.ncbi.nlm.nih.gov/pubmed/20516734
- Glioma Brain Cancer http://www.ncbi.nlm.nih.gov/pubmed/16899063
- Billary tract cancer http://www.ncbi.nlm.nih.gov/pubmed/19916793

Other researchers have also shown that hemp's cannabinoids are effective at treating Hodgkin's disease and Kaposi's Sarcoma. Hemp has also been proven to be effective in the treatment of alcohol abuse, ALS ("Lou Gehrig Disease"), arthritis, asthma, atherosclerosis, bipolar disorder, MRSA, depression, dystonia, epilepsy, hepatitis C, Parkinson's disease, psoriasis, sleep apnea, and anorexia nervosa.

TRANSFORMATION OF CONSCIOUSNESS?

In August of 2013, CNN's Chief Medical Correspondent and neurosurgeon, Dr. Sanjay Gupta, reversed his position on hemp's health benefits and even apologized for his previous stand against it. *"We have been terribly and systematically misled for nearly 70 years in the United States, and I apologize for my own role in that."*

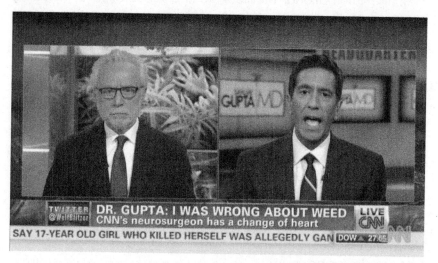

TWITTER @WolfBlitzer **DR. GUPTA: I WAS WRONG ABOUT WEED** LIVE CNN
CNN's neurosurgeon has a change of heart
SAY 17-YEAR OLD GIRL WHO KILLED HERSELF WAS ALLEGEDLY GAN DOW▲ 27.65

We were all lied to about the "dangers" of cannabis. A huge swath of our religious community was duped into perpetrating the myth that marijuana was a dangerous drug. Churches were infiltrated and co-opted in the campaign against this miraculous plant by creating the illusion that the plant's use was somehow immoral. It was a powerful tool to control the masses and unfortunately, most fell in line with this narrative. We bought into this thoughtform as well.

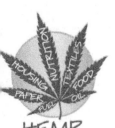

But how can a plant created by God be evil? When you step away from the powerful drug propaganda, you begin to see how absurd the claim has always been. This campaign makes personal the reality that the bigger the lie, the more believable it is. Claiming that cannabis was the "devil's weed" was a whopper and many good people, including us, got suckered!

Kudos to Dr. Gupta for having the intellectual integrity to review his entrenched medical bias against the plant and for going public with his new perspective on CNN: *"I apologize because I didn't look hard enough, until now,"* he said. *"I didn't look far enough. I didn't review papers from smaller labs in other countries doing some remarkable research, and I was too dismissive of the loud chorus of legitimate patients whose symptoms improved on cannabis."*

Gupta had previously taken the DEA at its word on the serious danger of addiction, which was never based on sound scientific proof. He was troubled when he found research predating the 1970 Controlled Substances Act (CSA) that classified cannabis as a schedule I controlled substance with *"a high potential for abuse."*

From Gupta: *"They didn't have the science to support that claim, and I now know that when it comes to marijuana neither of those things are true.* **It doesn't have a high potential for abuse, and there are very legitimate medical applications. In fact, sometimes marijuana is the only thing that works.**

Gupta continued: *"Take the case of Charlotte Figi, who I met in Colorado. She started having seizures soon after birth. By age 3, she was having 300 a week, despite being on seven different medications. Medical marijuana has calmed her brain, limiting her seizures to 2 or 3 per month. I have seen more patients like Charlotte first hand, spent time with them and come to the realization that it is irresponsible not to provide the best care we can as a medical community, care that could involve marijuana."*

POTENT PERSONAL PONTIFICATIONS

On The Robert Scott Bell Show, we have spotlighted numerous cases of families and children who benefit from the medicinal uses of hemp. While the medical literature supports a multitude of beneficial properties, it is critically important to bring those scientific revelations to life. Super Mom Penny Howard joined us to tell of her little girl, Harper Elle Howard, born April 12, 2010 and at just two weeks old, began having seizures. Over the course of 10 months, Harper traveled across the US and underwent a multitude of tests. In February 2011 she was diagnosed with a rare and in some cases life threatening genetic disorder known as CDKL5. Since then, CBD-rich hemp oil has reduced her seizure activity from over **three hundred** per day to **near zero**! http://www.hope4harper.com.

Moriah Barnhart joined us to talk about her experiences with CBD and medical marijuana. Her daughter has benefited tremendously while under medical treatment for a brain tumor. You can learn more about their story of extraordinary healing at http://dahliastrong.org and http://tinyurl.com/lwlu686.

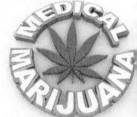

Renee Petro has been a vocal supporter of the growing medical marijuana movement in Florida. She wants it for her son Branden who suffers from frequent seizures. Since then, she's received praise and some skepticism — but what happened recently floored her. The Department of Children and Families (DCF) came knocking, launching an investigation from an anonymous tip. The claim was that Petro stopped giving her son his prescribed medicine and was instead giving him illegal cannabis. What do you think of this invasion of privacy and parental rights? We still have a long way to go to re-establish the legality of caring for children with this powerful, yet safe, medicinal plant. https://www.facebook.com/BrandenTheBrave

These super moms are getting together to spread the word about the healing benefits of hemp as the Cannamoms! Be sure to look out for the hashtag #cannamoms in social media to see what you can do to support the return of this miracle weed to its rightful place in our pantries. It's already in ours in the form of CBD-rich hemp oil **- legal in all 50 states!**

In 2011, my (RSB) wife, Nancy, had a tooth extracted. During the procedure, she sustained nerve damage and has since suffered with Trigeminal Neuralgia. We approached this new challenge with a multitude of natural remedies, from high dose fish oil to acupuncture with very little success. Out of desperation, she did resort to heavy prescription narcotics a couple of times, but only felt drugged with no change in the nerve pain whatsoever. One day, my good friend and colleague, Stuart Tomc, national educator for Nordic Naturals, brought HempMedsPX™ CBD-rich hemp oil to my attention. I immediately thought of the possible benefits for my wife. She tried it and after more than two years of suffering constant, unrelenting pain she found significant relief for the first time! It was a godsend! Along with body work from David Peterson at bodytuneupshop.com, she has become a functional human again, and for that I am truly grateful.

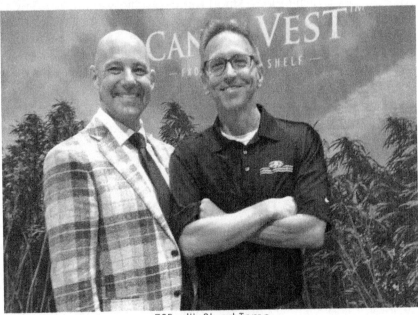

RSB with Stuart Tomc

We continue to be overwhelmed by uplifting stories of relief and recovery from so many people dealing with various ailments since going public with this information on radio. We pray that this information reaches all those in need of hemp's unique medicinal benefits, including the men and women serving in our armed forces who suffer serious depression and post traumatic stress disorder (PTSD). While we support all efforts and legislation to make medicinal marijuana available and free from recrimination, it's important to know that wherever you live in the United States, **YOU DON'T HAVE TO MOVE!**

The FDA does not want you to know that CBD from industrial hemp sold as a dietary supplement is available in all 50 states! So what can you do? Tell your local independent health foods store retailer that you want CBD and send them the link to Cannavest.com. Or call 1-855-758-7223 and get some directly.

Since the initial publication of *Unlock the Power To Heal*, the interest in cannabis as medicine has grown tremendously and is now legal in 23 states and the District of Columbia. The science of CBD is of particular interest to us, specifically because of its status as a dietary supplement, rather than a drug. This allows those who are in need to access the benefits of this extraordinary plant, even in the other 27 states where laws on cannabis have not yet changed. We owe much gratitude to **Stuart Tomc** for initially introducing us to reliable sources of quality CBD. He now serves as Vice President of Human Nutrition at Cannavest. We share Stuart's interest in scientific substantiation so that CBD's appropriate use will benefit the many who are in desperate need. His contributions to our growing understanding continue below:

CANNABIDIOL 101 – A PEEK INTO CANNABINOID CHEMISTRY

The endocannabinoid system (ECS) is a complex signaling network within the human body, that utilizes specialized lipid compounds, known as cannabinoids to control various physiological processes by interacting with various receptors (like lock and key) and regulatory enzymes. Cannabidiol (CBD) is often referred to as a "phytocannabinoid." Phytocannabinoids, of which well over 60 have been found to exist, are plant derivatives that contain a number of diverse chemical compounds that can affect appetite, metabolic health, pain sensation, inflammation/oxidative stress, thermoregulation, eye health, mood and memory. It's important to define phytocannabinoids as any plant-derived natural product capable of either—

1) directly interacting with cannabinoid receptors (CB1, CB2 or orphan receptor GPR55), or
2) sharing chemical similarity with cannabinoids that allow them to interact with other components of the ECS (e.g., enzymes that degrade and control cannabinoid levels, or
3) both.

CBD is the second most prominent compound found in the Cannabis sativa L. plant (the first is THC, tetrahydrocannabinol). Unlike THC, CBD can be legally purchased and used in all 50 states as a food product of agricultural hemp, is non-psychoactive (i.e. it does not result in feelings of euphoria) and appears to have a much broader range of medical applications. In particular, a recent review by Fernadez-Ruiz et al. concluded that CBD has beneficial effects on neurodegeneration, autoimmune disorders, heart and liver health. The mechanisms underpinning these effects are not well understood, but it is generally agreed upon that direct activation of CB1 and CB2 receptors (the primary targets of THC) do <u>not</u> explain the myriad of benefits from CBD administration. In fact, it has been reported that CBD affects a wide variety of ion channels:

- TRPV1
- TRPV2
- 5-HT3A
- TRPM8
- TRPA1

CBD may also influence the function of key receptors that are widely expressed and present throughout the body:

- GPR55
- PPARs
- 5-HT1A
- opioid
- glycine, etc.

Phytocannabinoids, and CBD in particular may also modulate a number of important enzymes:

- CYP1A1/2
- Mg-ATPase
- Fatty acid amide hydrolase
- MAGL
- 15-lipoxygenase
- Glutathione peroxidase

- Superoxide dismutase
- Catalase, etc.

They have also been know to affect cellular uptake processes, including but not limited to:
- adenosine and calcium uptake
- norepinephrine
- dopamine
- GABA
- 5-HT uptake
- choline uptake
- P-glycoprotein efflux, etc.

The mere existence of cannabinoid receptors throughout many tissues and organs of the human body, have mistakenly lead some enthusiasts to think that the Cannabis species/ Agricultural Hemp plant was intended to therapeutically (or recreationally) exploit the endocannabinoid system.

However, as nature is quite parsimonious this is simply a result of "biochemical serendipity" or "chemical coincidence" whereby the plant cannabinoids simply mimic our own. There are numerous examples of botanical compounds that have some homology or chemical similarity to other endogenous hormones (such as estrogen or androgen steroid hormones). We call these some of these compounds "phyto-estrogens" because although they are found in plants, they can interact with our own hormone receptors in humans. This scenario presents an opportunity to harness these plant derived natural products, or "Cannabis Chemistry" for optimizing human health, wellness and longevity via the endocannabinoid system.

As a result, CBD and other phytocannabinoids "talk" to just about every major organ system in the body, helping restore normal balance and physiologic homeostasis.

Nutritional scientists and applied physiologists remain enthusiastic to explore the potential to modulate physiologic systems in already healthy individuals. Some of these systems include: stress resilience, nervous system health, cardiometabolic health, recovery/ adaptation in physically active subjects, and immune system health.

Collectively, the ability of CBD to "talk" to multiple organ systems, combined with its remarkable safety profile and extremely low toxicity paint a bright future for this 5000 year old botanical superstar.

References:
- ✓ Fernandez-Ruiz J, et al. (2013). Cannabidiol for neurodegenerative disorders: Important new clinical applications for this phytocannabinoid? Br J Clin Pharmacol. 75(2): 323-333.
- ✓ Gertsch J, et al. (2010). Phytocannabinoids beyond the Cannabis plant do they exist? Br J Pharmacol. 160(3):523-9.
- ✓ Zias J, Stark H, Sellgman J, Levy R, Werker E, Breuer A, Mechoulam R. (1993) Early medical use of cannabis. Nature. 363(6426):215.
- ✓ De Petrocellis L and Di Marzo V (2010). Non-CB(1), Non-CB(2) receptors for endocannabinoids, plant cannabinoids, and synthetic cannabimimetics: focus on G-protein-coupled receptors and transient receptor potential channels. J Neuroimmune Pharmacol. 5:103–121.
- ✓ Raduner S, Majewska A, Chen JZ, Xie XQ, Hamon J, Faller B et al. (2006). Alkylamides from Echinacea are a new class of cannabinomimetics. Cannabinoid type-2 receptor-dependent and–independent immunomodulatory effects. J Biol Chem 281:S14192–S1S206.

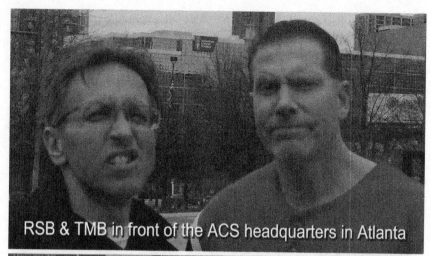

RSB & TMB in front of the ACS headquarters in Atlanta

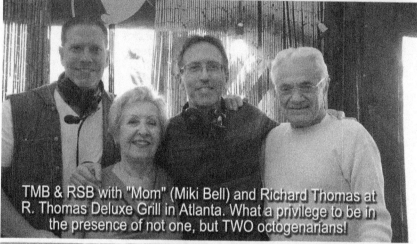

TMB & RSB with "Mom" (Miki Bell) and Richard Thomas at R. Thomas Deluxe Grill in Atlanta. What a privilege to be in the presence of not one, but TWO octogenarians!

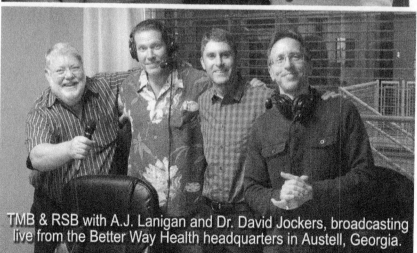

TMB & RSB with A.J. Lanigan and Dr. David Jockers, broadcasting live from the Better Way Health headquarters in Austell, Georgia.

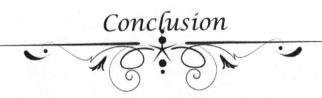

Conclusion

No one book is exhaustive in covering every aspect, technique and substance for healing. That would take a rather large library.

We brought together keys to unlock the basic starting points on your road to recovery and ultimate health maintenance. This information does not replace the assistance of appropriate (and preferably holistic) health care providers when needed, but it does provide a foundation upon which you may build a vibrantly healthy future – without anyone's permission.

Now go forth and tell everyone that you have the keys to **unlock the power to heal**. And please tell everyone you know to visit **www.UnlockThePowerToHeal.com**.

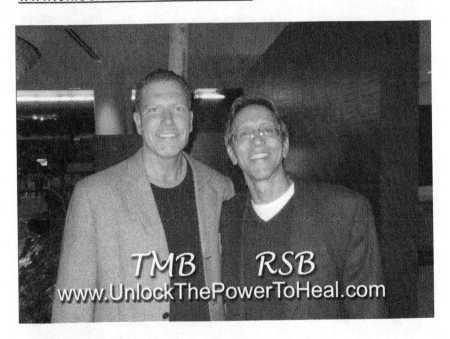

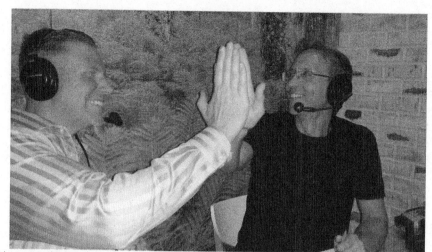

Above and Below – TMB, RSB, and the TTAC crew at the Vitality Bistro in Mt Dora, Florida

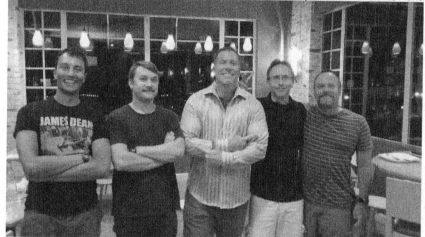

Below – TMB & Charlene present RSB with his Lifetime Achievement Award in Nashville (Dec 2015)

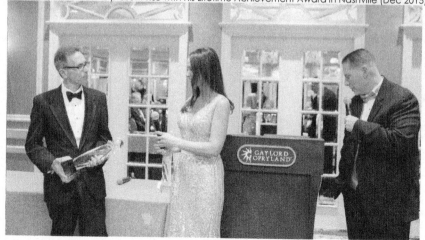

CPSIA information can be obtained
at www.ICGtesting.com
Printed in the USA
BVOW08s1644110118
504927BV00002B/123/P